D1565337

WHY BODYBUILDING FOR WOMEN?

Why not? Bodybuilding does not mean *just building* the body. The real meaning is remoulding or reshaping the body. Bodybuilding for women usually entails the use of weights to firm, reduce, build and shape a strong, healthy body of firm, svelte muscle-tissue that is outrageously feminine, curvy and attractive.

If you are thin, you can start by using extremely light weights so that you ease yourself into condition as the weeks go by. If you want to lose weight, you may be able to start with slightly heavier weights.

Remember *you* are in charge of the weights. *You* are using them as tools to sculpt *your* body to physical perfection.

With a proper diet, avoiding unhealthy habits, and a regular program of progressive bodybuilding, you can expect an improvement in:

- HEALTH
- FITNESS
- FIRMNESS, CURVACIOUSNESS AND WELL-BEING
- ENHANCED SELF-IMAGE AND CONFIDENCE

Remember—the benefits of *Bodybuilding. For Women* are too numerous, too exhilarating and too satisfying to pass up. You can start today!

BODY-BUILDING FOR WOMEN

Robert Kennedy

PUBLISHED BY POCKET BOOKS NEW YORK

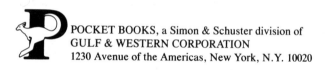
POCKET BOOKS, a Simon & Schuster division of
GULF & WESTERN CORPORATION
1230 Avenue of the Americas, New York, N.Y. 10020

CONTENTS

INTRODUCTION

Progressive resistance exercise apparatus, and more particularly "weights" (barbells and dumbells) are sometimes referred to as *iron pills*. Today doctors, scientists, coaches and physical educators are starting to understand fully the enormous capabilities and advantages that can be gained from the regular use of weights. It is pretty safe to assume that, if indeed weights *were* pills—they would be known as *miracle* working medicine. At times, it would seem that the benefits gained through their use *are* little short of miraculous.

I am asking you to believe in bodybuilding for women, via the use of progressive resistance exercise; that is, exercise that you can tailor to your own strength and condition. Weight training is the most popular and effective method of progressive resistance exercise.

You don't have to join the "grunt and groan brigade" to achieve results. Weight training can seem less physically demanding than many other forms of exercise, yet the movements are so concentrated that they effectively *command* your body to react under their authority.

Believe it! Modern weights can be used by you in the same way that a sculptor uses his hammer and chisel. Yes, you can sculpt and shape your body to your own specifications, adding a little bit here; taking a little off there. Male bodybuilders have been doing this successfully since the beginning of the century and today, the technique of shaping one's body through the systematic use of weights has become a well understood science. It is even claimed by some as an advanced *art* (*Pumping Iron,* Gaines and Butler).

Now it's the ladies' turn. Experts have discovered that although women cannot gain the large muscles of a Mr. Universe, nor the awesome definition which typifies the modern competitive male bodybuilder, they can in fact bring about change; and a more dramatic transformation would be hard to imagine.

Combining training techniques with nutritional plans, a healthy woman can remould her body to create the highly desired curvy feminine figure she may have dreamed impossible. You can gain or lose weight. You can add a new fitness and healthy condition. Aspiring women athletes can increase strength to aid their performance in any sport. Whatever your ultimate goal you will *feel* like a million dollars, and in the fastest possible time. Following the plan set down in this book, you will get to *look* even better.

BODY-BUILDING FOR WOMEN

I

BUT I DON'T WANT TO BE A WEIGHTLIFTER!

Ok! I can hear you. "But I don't want to be a Weightlifter." I've got news for you. Bodybuilding, weight training or pumping iron if you will, is *not weightlifting*. For clarification the following are the four categories of weight exercises:

1. Weightlifting

This is an Olympic sport in which one man (women don't participate internationally at present, but there's always a first time) competes against another in determining who lifts the heavier weight in a specific lift. Formal meets are held throughout the world and world championships are held annually.

Olympic lifting involves two lifts, *the snatch* (in which a barbell is raised from the floor to arm's length, above head, in one movement) and the *clean and jerk,* a movement whereby a weight is first lifted to the shoulders (cleaned) and then "thrown" to arm's length above head (jerked). Each competitor is allowed three attempts at each lift and the aggregate of his best *snatch* and his best *clean and jerk* go to make his *total* of the competition. The man who makes the best total wins the competition. Of course as in boxing and wrestling, there are weight classes.

2. Power lifting

Not a sport recognized by the Olympic Committee but nevertheless power lifting is becoming a true international sport. The lifts differ from the Olympic lifts in that they demand a higher degree of pure strength and perhaps a degree less explosive power and skill required by the Olympic movements.

There are three power lifts, the *bench press* which involves lying face up on a bench and pushing a barbell from the chest to arm's length; the *squat,* whereby a barbell is placed across the back of the shoulders and the individual lowers into a squatting position (or deep knee bend) returning to an upright stance; and the *dead lift,* where a barbell is raised from the floor until the lifter is in an upright position. Like the Olympic lifts there are weight classes. Three attempts on each lift are allowed, the best of each contributing towards the overall total.

Powerlifting, unlike Olympic lifting, has not proven an exclusive male sport. Women have invaded the ranks and today we have many great women powerlifters, some of whom regularly win *open* powerlifting competitions. That's right! Many of America's strongmen are being beaten in open competition—by stronger women!

3. Weight training

Alternatively known as *pumping iron, bodybuilding* or *progressive resistance exercise.* This is the use of weights as "tools" to add health and strength for sports or even more commonly to remould and shape the human body. In weight *training* there are no efforts at "jerking" the weight to an overhead position, nor any teeth clenching efforts to lift the most weight possible. Weight training involves steady flowing movements or "repetitions" using barbells and dumbells to increase resistance and concentrate the effect. Now, you could one day *want* to be a weightlifter or power lifter. Or you may wish to use weights for strength training to help you improve in a particular sport. I have devoted a special chapter to these specialized fields. The majority of women reading this book are probably interested in improving their bodies, and would welcome the fringe benefit of dynamic health and fitness.

No, you don't have to be a weight*lifter* because the only relationship between weight *lifting* and weight *training* is that similar apparatus is used. Everything else is different.

Why bodybuilding for women?

Why not? Men have monopolized so many aspects of life that women have almost felt guilty about thinking of participating. Well, bodybuilding is no longer for men alone. The name itself is slightly misleading. Bodybuilding, whether applied to men or women, does not mean just *building* the body.

The real meaning is *remoulding* or *reshaping* the body. Many overweight men who take up bodybuilding find that in their case it is *body reducing*. The same of course, applies to women. Bodybuilding for women

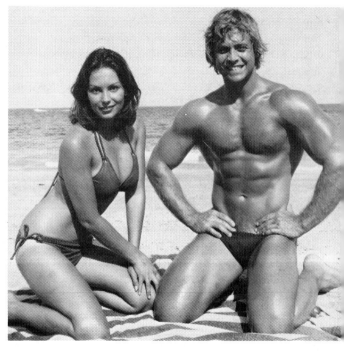

Bodybuilders Pattie Cella and John Kemper are examples of what can be achieved by sensible exercise habits and scientific nutrition. (Photo: Falcon)

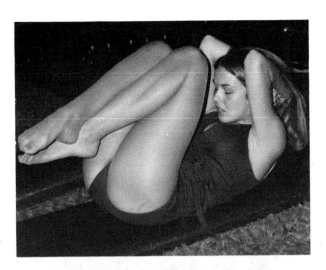

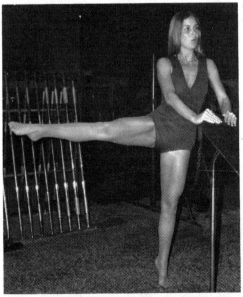

Sandy Nista, daughter of Noe Nista (a multi-winner and owner of Nista's Gym. Cerritos, California) has been an ardent bodybuilder since her teens. (Photo: Bill Reynolds Photos)

usually entails the use of weights to firm, reduce, build and shape a strong, healthy body of firm, svelt muscletissue that is outrageously feminine, curvy and attractive.

The beauty of weights is that you can *tailor* the resistance to your condition. In other words, if you are painfully thin and weak, you can start by using extremely light weights so that you ease yourself into condition as the weeks go by. As you get stronger and fill out, you will be able to add a little more weight to the bar. Gradually you will ease yourself into the kind of shape and condition you've always wanted.

Women who are on the large end of the scale or are more athletic, may be able to start with slightly heavier weights, but even so, as a beginner to weight training you should be prepared to start in "light." Be content to make haste slowly. There is little sense in trying to see how much you can lift when you first get into bodybuilding. This can lead to pulled muscles or minor strains, and ultimately missed workouts, dejection and confusion.

Remember *you* are in charge of the weights. *You* are using them as tools to sculpt *your* body to physical perfection. The moment you start trying to lift huge barbells that prove too much for your present strength you are putting yourself in a secondary "out of charge" position. The weight is king instead of you.

To get back to the original question, "Why Bodybuilding for Women?" Isn't the market saturated with diet courses, exercise routines and new super exercise gadgets, all claiming to "re-make your figure in double-quick time"? One only has to go to the local drug store to find all types of "so called" diet pills, drinks and mixes designed to "take off" pounds. Open a magazine or newspaper and you will be deluged with articles showing the latest slim-and-trim discoveries. Every other page is devoted to ads offering answers to your physical deficiencies.

What is the most often used topic of conversation apart from the weather and the state of the country? Right—*Diet and exercise*. So why another book on exercise? *Bodybuilding for Women* yet! A book which has the audacity to recommend dastardly things like weights, barbells, dumbells; paraphernalia that reeks of YMCA and all the macho muscle 'n sweat that goes with it.

The answer is, and I'll only say it *once* here (in the hope that you appreciate that I would like to write it across the sky in mile high letters). THIS BOOK ON WEIGHT TRAINING FOR WOMEN EXISTS BECAUSE THE AUTHOR HAS CONCLUDED AFTER 23 YEARS OF CONCENTRATED RESEARCH ON THE SUBJECT, THAT WEIGHT TRAINING IS THE MOST EFFECTIVE METHOD TO SHAPE THE FEMALE BODY.

I do concede that cardio-vascular fitness is best stimulated by jogging or skipping. I will also admit that diet education plays an enormous role in the end result of any exercise program. Both will be discussed at length later. But where a person wants to remould and firm up *every* area of her body nothing is more effective than weights. Stay with us.

II

YOUR REWARDS

I won't claim that progressive resistance exercises will improve every aspect of your existence, but when combined with the scientific nutritional plan outlined later, the results are little short of miraculous!

"Ok," you demand, "just what can those ugly uncouth-looking weights do for me?"

If figure consciousness has kept you from enjoying dancing, swimming, tennis or anything else, then a new figure achieved by my proven methods could mean a whole new world of enjoyment for you. Even the most pleasurable physical act—lovemaking—can be marred by self consciousness. Thousands upon thousands of women would rather forego the pleasures of sexual intercourse than reveal an out-of-condition body to the man they want. Better, they rationalize, to remain dressed and be *thought* unattractive than to undress and remove all doubt. You may be one of the victims of this unwelcome body self-consciousness.

Now the good news: Weight training combined with a thermodynamically balanced food intake can change your shape faster than any other method known. Exactly how this is achieved is explained in later chapters.

Right now you may only be concerned with improving your appearance. Most of us are. In fact, it's hard to even consider the benefits of working and achieving positive *good* health, especially when we are not actually suffering *bad* health. But being healthy *is* important. It helps you, not only survive the events of the day, but it gives you the greatest chance of actually enjoying it.

Regular exercise doesn't *automatically* give an ill person health, but it *does* help to secure and promote dynamic health in the able-bodied. True robust health is your God-given heritage. Most of us start out life with our full share. It is up to you to maintain it. The noted medical author, Franklin P. Adams wrote: "Health is the thing that makes you feel that *NOW* is the best time of the year."

With a proper diet, avoiding unhealthy habits, and a regular program of progressive exercise movements, you can "fix" your health at a dynamic "high" which only bad luck can take away.

Aside from normal good health there is an added plus—fitness. It is a near euphoric condition that *comes* almost automatically to the active child. It *stays* with the adolescent active in sports, but *leaves* most of us when we take up the responsibility of earning a living. But it can be brought back with the sensible training program I advocate. When did you last know fitness? When were you last feeling so light footed that you wanted to run up a flight of stairs three at a time?

When did you last yearn to run from the office or even *to* the office. True fitness is based on the ability of the heart and lungs to cope with extended exertion. When you have it, you want to move.

When you don't you've lost something important. What an unfortunate man was poor Paul Terry, who loved to brag, "When I feel like exercising, I just lie down until the feeling goes away." Dare to be different! If you promise yourself today to follow the principles outlined in this book you will receive a bonus—a better self-image.

Many men and women today suffer from some form of neurosis. It *slips* into our lives with modern living; and *zooms* through the door where there is a void of love or an absence of meaningful work. Neurosis can result in part from a poor self-image, triggered by disgust or shame with one's physical condition. They say you can tell a man with dirty socks by the look on his face. Perhaps your unhappiness is caused by *your* dissatisfaction with *your* body and condition. Isn't it reasonable then, to expect that, with an improvement in health, fitness, firmness, curvaciousness and well-being that your self image and confidence will also improve?

What are the benefits of bodybuilding for women? Whatever they prove to be in your case, they are too numerous, too exhilarating and too satisfying to pass up.

GETTING MOTIVATED

Exercise is boring. Why kid ourselves? Perhaps progressive resistance exercise is less boring than the more static "movements" of yoga, isometrics or even calisthenics, but nevertheless it is all "rather a bore." So why on Earth am I recommending regular exercise for the rest of your days? Simply because what *boring exercise* can do for you is *the most exciting* experience

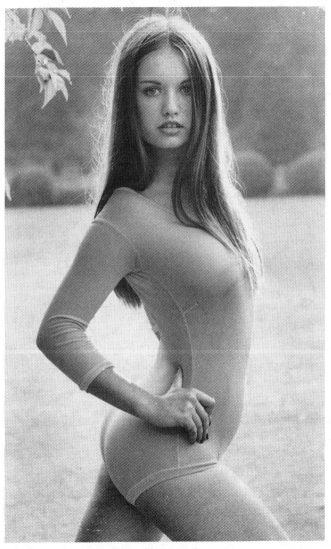

"New Breed" bodybuilder is Georgie Steer of South Africa. She supplements her regular workouts with gymnastic training.

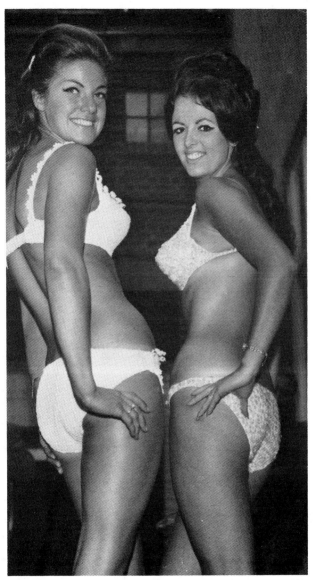

Kathleen Winstanley and Pat Wheeldon both use progressive bar-bell training.

of all. It's a woman's (or man's) best means of achieving good health, shape and an energetic, productive life. Consequently it is worth your time to try and make the best of potentially tedious training. The essayist Frank Knox wrote: "I have never suffered from boredom. Life is much too interesting if one attacks it with vigor." Perhaps you have not always been so successful in keeping boredom at bay. I certainly have not. However, Knox spoke simple truth. Boredom can be beaten, if you stand your ground and open the attack. Don't wait around for something to happen. Just get out of that chair—and *start* that exercise. Overcome any lack of willingness to "take a workout" by simply—beginning.

Glenn Swengros, the director of program development of the President's Council on Physical Fitness wrote in his book, *Fitness with Glenn Swengros* (Hawthorn Book Inc., N.Y.) a nine part formula for beating the training blues. Here they are in essence:

1. Make an honest appraisal of what you hope to attain. Convince yourself of the importance of your workouts. Know why you are exercising and how each part of your body is affected.
2. Do not make your workout routine too difficult, or too long. Set realistic goals.
3. Make sure that the area where you choose to work out is well lighted and adequately ventilated. Small, stuffy basements do not make an ideal training area.
4. Take measurements of height, weight, hips, thighs, waist and any other problem areas. In fact, it's worth noting all measurements. Just for the record. Record the date too. Chart your progress as the weeks roll by.

5. Play music while you exercise. Try to co-ordinate the repetitions with the rhythm of the music. Although not a necessity, nor always possible, music does make the workout go faster, as well as more enjoyably.
6. When you don't feel like exercising, force yourself to get started. Afterwards you will feel invigorated and glad you went ahead.
7. Persuade a friend to exercise with you. You might even talk your "better half" into joining you (if you can get him enthusiastic over improving his physical shape).
8. Television can be used as a backdrop in some cases. Many T.V. shows do not command 100% concentration, yet they can relieve the boredom of "going it alone."
9. Keep an eye out for new locations. You don't always have to exercise in the bedroom or down in the basement. You can perform some of your workout in the living room or even outside when weather permits. If you exercise at a gym, then consider changing gyms if you find things are getting humdrum.

If you are sick, have a headache, or a cold, forget your workout. But don't kid yourself that you are *too tired to exercise* when all you are suffering from is a bout of laziness. I have found the best way to get into a workout on those "listless" days is to start with a little rope jumping. This will get the heart beating a little faster, your blood coursing more vigorously—and presto—you are rarin' to go.

In my own experience, it is always harder to resist an armchair after a substantial meal. Try to get your workout "in" *before* eating. Above all, remember that you are training so that come next season you are going to look and feel like a billion bucks of super femininity. You're going to have the kind of curves and fit-for-anything-condition that not even a suit of armor could hide.

And wow! When you step out on that beach, you better be ready! If it's bikini weather, you'd better have an escort. If you don't you're going to find scores of enthusiastic applicants for the job.

III

THOSE LOVELY WOMEN OF IRON

Ok! You say—just tell me about a few prominent or luscious women who have benefited from lifting weights.

A large percentage of women beauty contest winners train regularly with iron. Take *Bridget Gibbons* of Lancashire, England. "People thought I was a bit of a freak when I first started using weights. They told me I'd become muscle-bound. I must admit I was a bit worried myself since I didn't know much about it then. But women don't build up huge veined muscles like men, when they use weights, and it's marvelous for the figure. I am sure millions of women around the world would try weights if they knew what I know." Bridget has been training since 1976. She does her workouts at the Bolton Health Club. Ken Heathcote who runs the club says: "She lifts heavier weights than a lot of the men. It's a question of determination really."

Bridget won the prestigious N.A.B.B.A. (Miss Universe Contest in London) and was runner up in the Miss World Contest. The man behind her training is boyfriend Gordon Pasquill, a bodybuilder. They often work out side by side.

Miss Europe and Miss Body Beautiful U.S.A., *Jacqueline Nubret* is an ardent weight trainer. "Jackie" lives in Paris, is a lawyer and is married appropriately to Serge Nubret, a Mr. Universe winner. She trains three times a week using both dumbells and barbells, eats pretty much what she wants. When she has a guest spot or a contest, she reduces her carbohydrates to a minimum for two or three weeks prior to the date. "It may seem paradoxical," says Jackie, "but pumping iron has given me my feminine curves and gracefulness."

Natalie Kahn, whose husband is Bob Packer, the AAU Coach for the US powerlifting team, says of weightlifting: "It's given me self confidence in everything. The stronger I get, the more things I feel I can do outside of weightlifting. I'm more outspoken too. Bob says I'm getting more arrogant every day."

Former gymnast *Linda Cheeseman,* of Wakefield, England turned to weights to improve her body. She too is one of Europe's top beauty contestants, having won a room full of trophies at National and International levels. Linda is ladies' editor for Physical Fitness and Beauty for one of Europe's top health magazines. She never exercises less than three times a week with the iron pills.

Queen of American weight training is lovely *Vera Christensen* of Florida. She has been writing about barbells and dumbells and their connection with female beauty and curves for over twenty years. Herself, a complete example of physical perfection and fitness, Vera has been hoisting Iron two or three hours

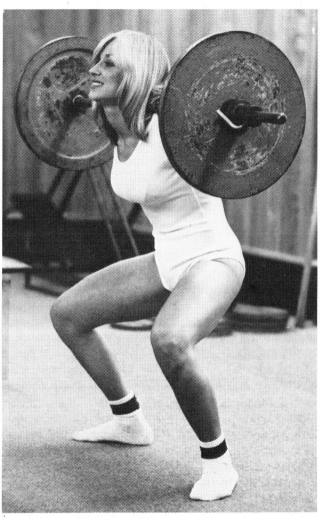

Top beauty contestant Bridget Gibbons exercises hard with weights several times a week.

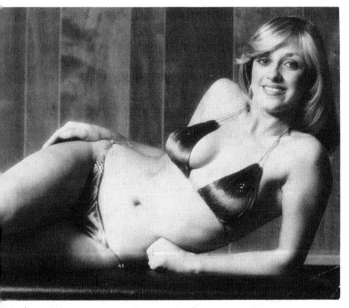

Bridget Gibbons again, just being beautiful.

a week all her adult life. "Barbells and dumbells are the nearest thing to a youth pill," says Vera. "My husband and I have always used them and the results in body shape, strength and fitness have *never* been disappointing."

In the film world both *Marilyn Monroe* and *Jayne Mansfield* used weights to add curves to their figures. Before her fatal car accident Jayne measured a beautiful 40-22-38. Publicity figures at the time had her waist at 18 with a bustline measurement of 42. This put her waist smaller than her husband Mickey Hargitay's upper arm. Not so.

Mickey Hargitay was a former Mr. Universe winner who met Jayne when he was in Mae West's *Muscle Review* back in the early 60's. *Mae West* herself was always a great believer in weight training and even in her "eighties" she would get out her silver dumbells and go through a few light movements to preserve tone and shape.

Racquel Welch not only watches her diet carefully but she also exercises regularly with weights. Because of this training she has maintained strong limbs, young looking muscles and a firmness seldom found on women half her age. "I enjoy being healthy," says Racquel, "and looking after one's body on a daily basis is just as important as cleaning one's teeth or bathing. Health, shape and fitness are at the top of my list."

Sally Field, who changed her image from T.V.'s "Flying Nun" to one of a dynamic, intelligent actress, also works with weights to keep her body fabulous!

Yes, the list is endless. Suddenly the new secret method is out. The public is discovering weights. Bodybuilding for women is here to stay. If it works for so many big names, think what it will do for you!

There's also a long list of women athletes who use weights. In fact, it is pretty safe to say that most

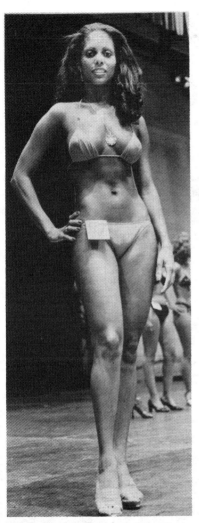
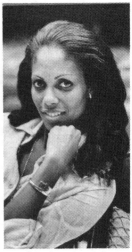

Jacqueline Nubret, a Paris lawyer and wife of Mr. Universe, Serge Nubret.

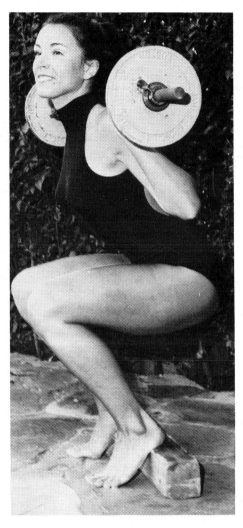

Beauty editor, international title winner, and accomplished gymnast, Linda Cheeseman has worked out with barbells and dumbells for 15 years.

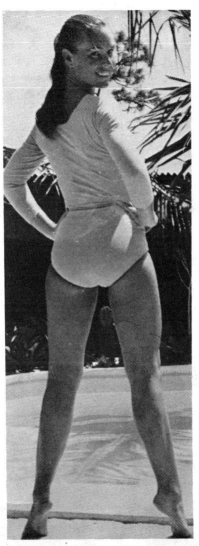

Vera Christensen of Florida has been training with weights for a quarter of a century. She is women's editor of STRENGTH AND HEALTH MAGAZINE.

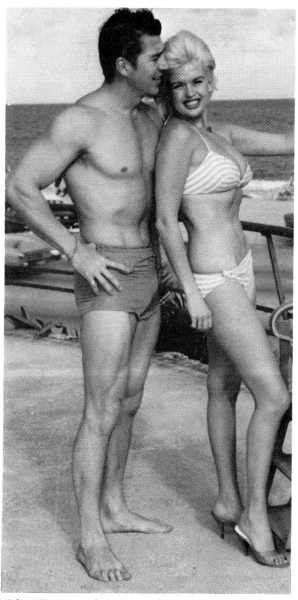

Mickey Hargitay and Jayne Mansfield set the world on fire with their weight trained bodies and whirlwind marriage.

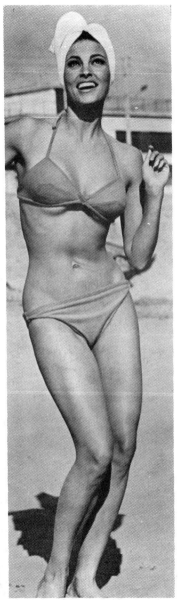

Racquel Welch always keeps fit, firm, and healthy. She believes in regular and vigorous exercise and a sound nutrition program.

women training seriously for an Olympic medal find weights *necessary* to retain their fullest muscle tone and body power.

In the tennis world there's *Margaret Court,* whose coach Frank Sedgman put her through hours of training with weights. Her iron workouts speeded up her game, enabled her to handle her racquet with greater ease and precision; and improved her flexibility and strength. Her Wimbledon championship title proved it.

Marathon runner *Pat Connors* began weight training to improve endurance. She accomplished this and now maintains her basic strength with regular weight-training.

Mary Peters, women's pentathlon Olympic champion, has used heavy weights in training for a dozen years. Her coach, Robert McShane, explained: "Mary loves the ecstasy involved in the intensely hard work and fierce concentration. And when it's all over there is profound relief, pride and joy at having endured so much, so well, for so long."

Coach *Mary Darin* of the Madison, Wisc. Y.M.C.A. agrees, "It's like winning a race all over again; the promise of a trim, fit body gets most people interested in weight training. But there is much more; even promises you don't dare to make to yourself are fulfilled. Not only do you find the physical benefits, but unexpected mental boosts."

Powerlifter *Terry Dillard* competes for the Iowa Lakes Community College in AAU contests. She had actually set an Iowa record for men and women in the 114 pound class, with a squat lift of 225 pounds, almost double her bodyweight. Terry has acquired a figure that not only rates with the best around, but one that exudes a quiet strength, stature and health that calisthenics alone could not produce.

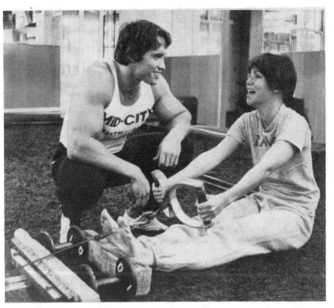

Sally Field gets some tips from the world's most successful physical culturist, Arnold Schwarzenegger.

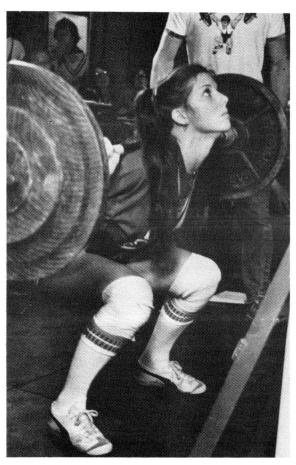

Terry Dillard, holder of several powerlifting records. (Photo: Wide World)

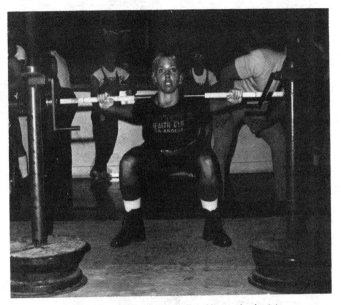

Carol Connors of California enjoys her film and television career,
yet still finds time to train and compete in powerlift meets.

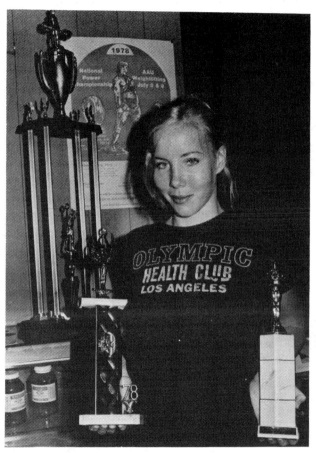

Carol with a *few* of her awards.

Rosalyn Drexler, novelist, playwright, professional wrestler and amateur powerlifter, comments, "The Iron game is a beautiful risk. In a split second, one can lose everything or be brought closer to the essential delight of existence."

Blond haired, blue-eyed *Carol Connors* won her first AAU Powerlift competition in 1978. She squatted 195 pounds, bench pressed 120 pounds, and dead lifted 260 pounds. Lifting against 8 other men and women in her division, she set two new Cal State records and won the Schwarz formula trophy (formula for comparing body-weight to total poundage lifted). Carol is seen regularly by 10 million viewers on Chuck Barris' NBC's "Gong Show" in which she is the regular announcer.

One of the first women to popularize modern weight training was *"Pudgy" Evill Stockton,* of California. Ms. Stockton involved herself in all aspects of weight training and weight lifting throughout the 1940's and 50's. Magazines such as Bob Hoffman's *Strength and Health* delighted in reporting her exploits with barbells. "Pudgy" would lift for fun, competition, or for her own personal achievement. Weights were her love. Still are. At her best she could deadlift 300 pounds, raise a dumbell of 90 pounds above her head with one hand and "snatch lift" 150 pounds.

IV

EVALUATING YOUR PRESENT CONDITION

How fit are you right now? How fat are you? Are you underweight? Are you healthy?

Very few people indeed are in touch with their physical condition or their physical appearance. If you asked a *fit* person what type of condition he was in, you may well get the answer, "Lousy, I need more exercise." On the other hand, you could ask a totally *unfit* person the same question and get a resounding, "fit as a fiddle!"

If you are in doubt about your present appearance, try the *mirror test*. Get all your clothes off and stand in front of a full length mirror. Turn all the lights on. Do this at a time when you are completely alone. You don't want any distractions. Cast your eyes across your shoulders, look at your arms, chest, waistline; take in your hips, upper legs and calves. Check your overall proportions. Are your lower legs big enough?

Have you too much weight on the upper outer thigh area? Is there fat around your lower back? Are your upper arms a lot thicker near the shoulders than they are near the elbow? Now try to decide what you want to correct. Is your posture good? Are you underweight—or is fat your enemy?

The surest way of finding out if you are carrying too much fat under your skin is to try the *pinch test* (medically known as the skinfold test).

Simply pinch some of your skin between your thumb and forefinger. Best sites are the triceps (back of the upper arm), side of waist, top of thigh or side of chest. If your pinched skin is more than half an inch this is an indication that you are carrying too much fat.

Remember, fat is a *killer* of shape. It fills in the areas where one muscle curves into another. Fat "spoils" the natural curve running from the waist to the hips. It *destroys* the descending silhouette from the hips to the knees. There should not be a mound of fat on the upper, outer thigh. The knees, together with the ankles and wrists, should always be bony and virtually devoid of fat. This boniness in the legs particularly dramatizes the curves of the thigh and calf muscles. Superfluous fat in the knee and ankle area will give your leg a straight *uninteresting* appearance.

Fat will *kill* your cleavage. Whereas fat on the upper chest area will inevitably increase the size of your breasts and certainly your bustline measurement, it will also act to nullify the appearance of your bosom. Why? Because the appeal of your breasts depends not on size, but on *delineation*. If your breasts show a definite point where they can be seen to rise from the sternum then they will have the glandular beauty that nature intended. However, should your entire bosom area be coated with adipose tissue (fat) then your breasts will not have that almost inexplicable yet unde-

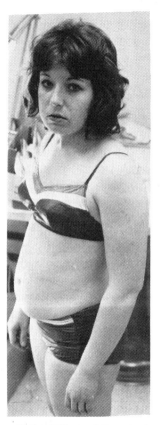

Cathy Miller, of Canada, transformed her body in five weeks using the principles advocated in this book. (Before)

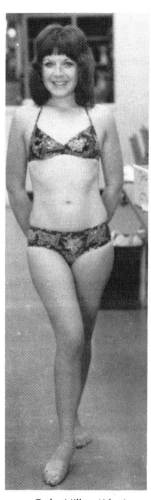

Cathy Miller. (After)

niable magic attractiveness. You will simply appear to have two gently rising "hills" on your upper chest as opposed to a pair of sensuous feminine breasts.

One way of finding out about how you look is to have someone take a few quick Polaroid pictures of you in the "buff." Within a minute or two you will be able to sit down and closely scrutinize your physical condition. You can even compare yourself with pictures of women noted for their great bodies in magazines or newspapers, or with earlier pictures of yourself. The important thing is that you become *totally aware* of how good or bad you look. Learn about yourself. Try to determine what your ideal weight should be. Find out exactly how much fat you have on your legs, hips, waist, shoulders. Keep aware of your physical appearance and half the battle is won.

It may be harder to evaluate your physical fitness. Obviously if you can run up a few flights of stairs without being unduly out of breath, then you are probably pretty fit. On the other hand, if you feel bad just walking a block or two then you are in trouble.

Whatever your own personal feelings are towards your current fitness level, it is strongly recommended that you ask your doctor to arrange a physical stress test. Tell him (or her) the type of exercise you'll be undertaking. Show your doctor this book by all means. It is always advisable before undertaking any type of exercise or nutrition program, to have a complete medical checkup. You will find that a stress test can be fun (you will probably have to step up and down on some boxes or jog on a machine while your breathing and pulse rate are monitored). After you get the "go ahead" from your doctor, you'll be thrilled that you have a clean bill of health.

Alternatively should an irregularity be uncovered,

you're still ahead, because you can take steps to correct any malfunction brought to light by the testing.

Whatever you do, resist the temptation suddenly to throw yourself into a furious session of formal exercise. Remember we are going to *coax,* not *pound* your body into a new dynamic sensual shape. We do not want you to be hampered by exercise "aches and pains" because you neglected to take the advice given here. Your new body will assuredly come—but to do the job right follow the steps; and start at the beginning.

THE AGE FACTOR

Men usually find the call to bodybuilding comes between the ages of 16 to 19. The reason is simple. They are tired of being skinny and laughed at. Women, on the other hand, often start to exercise only when they see a deterioration in their condition. This usually begins when they first notice those dreaded signs of adipose tissue—fat!

Thousands of men take up bodybuilding to lose flab, and untold numbers of skinny women want to add flesh to their limbs. However, the fact remains. Most ladies undertake a program of formal exercise for one reason. To *lose* excess weight.

Many of these women will be asking the question: Is it too late? Am I too old? The amusing thing (to me, not to them) is that I have been asked this question not just by people in their 40's, 50's, 60's and 70's, but by people in their 20's and 30's. And even in their teens!

To quote the greatest living bodybuilding authority of all, Oscar Heidenstam (*Modern Bodybuilding,* Emerson Books Inc., N.Y.) "There is no exact age at which to start bodybuilding. You can be a teenager, middle-aged or elderly." All you have to do is follow the advice of this book carefully and tailor the exercises to your present condition and needs. The urge to get into shape can hit you at any stage in life, and age does not automatically disqualify you.

As I mentioned earlier you should get a medical evaluation of your condition before starting any diet or exercise program. Another thing to remember is (fit or unfit, old or young) begin your bodybuilding schedule gently. *Never* start with heavy weights. Never work till exhaustion; never strain to life your limit and last but not least; never exercise before warming up the body completely.

Bodybuilding is not a dangerous sport. But weight training involves exercises which are completely outside the range of everyday muscular movements. And therefore, hear these words: *Train don't strain*. Coax your muscles to fitness and beauty. Teenagers will easily adapt to the different bodybuilding movements. But if you are older, your musculature may be just a bit less responsive. Take it easy—and this also applies if you trained progressively in the past but haven't done so in a few years. Start S-L-O-W-L-Y and watch for top, uninterrupted results.

V

BODYBUILDING PRINCIPLES

Don't get scared. There's nothing particularly difficult about bodybuilding. Few can assimilate everything at once, so keep this book handy, and refer back to it when you need to.

There are four distinctly different aims in bodybuilding. Weight training can help "fatties" who want to slim and "skinnies" who want to build up, the "unfit" who want to get fitter, as well as the person seeking more strength for whatever reason. The key factor in whether you want to build up or tear down is not so much in your choice of exercises, though these will vary somewhat, but more in the amount of calories you ingest. Details on this later.

How often should you work out? Weight training is an extremely concentrated form of exercise. It is therefore almost a universal law that you only train every other day, allowing a complete day's rest from "lifting" after each session. Most practitioners of the iron game train Mondays, Wednesdays and Fridays, allowing themselves a "free" day after each workout, and of course a two day rest at the weekend. You may of course train Tuesdays, Thursdays and Saturdays, or Wednesdays, Fridays and Sundays if you wish. The point is that training three times a week is *enough*. More may overtire you, especially at the onset. There is no advantage in taking more than the recommended dosage of "iron pills." Weight training tears down cellular tissue during exercise, and it requires the following day to re-build; otherwise you may find yourself overtired, listless and dejected from "overtraining."

Training with a Mirror

If possible, exercise in front of a mirror. Seeing yourself go through the movements is recommended for several reasons.

1. You can see exactly how you are doing keeping arms level, head up, posture correct, etc.
2. There is a new dimension to the exercise area. You are more aware of training with yourself. Shorter rests between exercises will result along with a greater awareness and enthusiasm for completing the workout.
3. You will become more familiar with your body, noticing the parts of your body that need attention, where you could use less weight or more muscle, better carriage or poise.
4. A mirror helps to ward off feelings of claustrophobia if your training area is at all tight.
5. Seeing yourself in the mirror repeatedly will help you to acquire proper co-ordination and to concentrate on what you are doing.

Do Not eat a heavy meal before training

Vigorous exercise not only makes you feel uncomfortable after a large meal, it is also ill-advised. Digestion is best during completely inactivity. Physical exertion impedes it. Try to wait at least two hours after a big meal before your workout.

When is the best time to train?

There is no preferred time to exercise. It's a matter of when you can best fit it into your work and family commitments.

The important thing (although not absolutely essential) is that you try to train at the same time each exercise day. This will tend to "set" your internal clock and after a few weeks your body will actually start to look forward to your workouts, energizing itself for exertion at the accustomed time.

What are "sets" and "reps"?

Sets and reps (repetitions) are two phrases which you have to make yourself familiar with, not just because this book uses them but because they are the fundamental terminology of weight training.

When you perform an exercise, say for ten counts and then replace the weights on the floor for a breather, that is known as one "set." These counts or repetitions are known as "reps." If you do three sets of twelve reps, that is usually written as 3 x 12. Two sets of fifteen repetitions will appear as 2 x 15.

How long do I rest between sets?

This depends on the exercise. If you have just finished a vigorous set of squats (considered one of the more strenuous movements, because it involves the large muscles of the legs and hips) then you will probably require a good minute or two to recover your breath before performing another set. On the other hand, some exercises are considerably less tiring and you may need only twenty seconds or so before you are ready for the next set. A usual guide as to when you are ready for a subsequent set is when your breathing returns to normal.

How much weight do I use?

The golden rule here is to start very light. No two people use exactly the same poundages in all their exercises. You are the best judge of the amount of weight to use for each movement yourself. Stay well within your strength. You should never be straining or jerking the weight up. Suggested starting poundages are listed with each exercise; however, you may use slightly more or even less, depending on your current strength, condition, potential, age and individual tolerance to progressive resistance exercise.

Remember that of foremost importance is the *correct* performance of each exercise over its full range of movement. Bear in mind that a given weight may seem positively light during the first few repetitions yet prove to be quite an effort to lift during the last few reps.

Once you have gotten fully accustomed to handling barbells and dumbells and can perform the exercises correctly for eight, ten or twelve repetitions then you may find it gratifyingly easy to add 5 pounds or more to the weight used. However, only when you can perform an exercise for the recommended number of repetitions should you add weight to the bar.

If you decide to train in the company of other

women, you will find that some people will be handling more weight than others, even though their experience, weight, age and measurements may be almost identical. This is just nature at work.

Some people are naturally stronger than others. It may be a matter of bone lengths, leverage, tendon structure, temperament and untold (unseen) other advantages. We are all different, but even when we appear almost identical there can still be that unknown factor which makes one woman stronger or more energetic than another.

Dr. Herbert M. Shelton (*Exercise,* Natural Hygiene Press) wrote: "Caution must be used not to carry the exercise to the point of fatigue, nervous depletion or circulatory embarrassment. If exercise is followed by trembling, fainting, excessively difficult breathing, blueness of lips or extremities, or prolonged fatigue, it has been carried too far. Except in cases where great endurance is desired, exercise should not be prolonged beyond a slight feeling of fatigue."

Is there a special way to breathe during exercise?

There is a recommended way to breathe during vigorous progressive exercise. Quick gulps; in most cases one breath for each repetition. Deep breathing increases the amount of oxygen you make available to the lungs to circulate in the blood stream. Generally, your body will be a guide as to how much oxygen you need. Some exercises such as squats (heavy movement) make a large demand on your oxygen supply. Other less strenuous movements will require less oxygen. Your job is to supply the demand for air without interfering with the comfort or execution of the exercise.

Also, it is senseless to take in more air than is

needed. In fact, this practice known as hyperventilation could lead to dizziness. But it is essential that adequate oxygen is supplied. Your job is to provide a regular balanced air intake. Not too much; not too little. Breathing through the nose is often advocated in light exercises such as yoga and easy calisthenics; however, in weight training, it is far better to gulp in air through the mouth. It is quicker and you can take in more. Let the air out through somewhat puckered lips. This controls the outflow and allows the lungs to deflate in an organized manner. Breathing correctly during your workout also serves a second purpose. It acts as a pacer for your repetitions, helping the general control flow of each lifting movement.

It is often a good idea to breathe deeply after each set of repetitions. Fill the lungs from top to bottom, until you can breathe in no longer. Exhale slowly. Correct breathing, according to Oscar Heidenstam, "Can improve your posture and mould the bust. It will brighten your complexion and give you a feeling of general well-being." It is not generally realized that breathing is the most important function of the human body. You can do without food, water, sleep, or exercise for several days, but stop breathing for five minutes and that's it. Hello heaven!

The nose is a fine filter for dust and germs, but since you will be breathing through your mouth when training, it is obviously important to select a clean, dust-free training area. Best of all of course, is to train in an area which has a comfortable flow of *fresh* air.

The general rule for breathing during an exercise is: Breathe *in* just before beginning the repetition and breathe *out* in a controlled manner as you complete the hardest part of the exercise. For example, if you are "pressing" (pushing up) a weight overhead from the shoulders, then breathe *in* just before starting the push and breathe *out* as the weight gets past the hard part and your elbows lock out with the poundage overhead. Remember—one breath for each repetition.

What about warming up?

A good jockey "warms up" his horse before a race. He gives him a little light work before the run and never takes his horse directly from the stable into the race. After the event, he gradually lessens the speed and walks his horse around for awhile. Few weight trainers, male or female, show as much intelligence or concern for their own bodies. It would be laughable if it were not so serious a matter—but I have seen people carefully warm up their *cars,* then drive to the gym and rush into a heavy workout—with no attempt at warming up their bodies.

Fewer injuries are sustained by those who spend a few minutes doing very light exercise before their workouts. A couple of minutes jumping rope or running in place will get the heart pumping, your blood coursing, and you'll be "fired up" for your workout. It is also a good idea to go through the general movements of your workout with very light weights or even no weights at all. As further protection your first set of any exercise should always be done with an extremely light weight. This warms up the tendons, joints and muscle tissue, avoiding the undue stress and strain of training at full pelt with "cold" muscles. As Arnold Schwarzenegger says in his excellent book, *Education of a Bodybuilder* (Simon and Schuster), "Give your body a chance to adjust to the new activity. It's a way of saying to the body, 'I'm giving you a warm-up now, take your time, fall into it easily. In a few minutes I'm going to hit you hard!' "

LAYING OFF TRAINING FOR A WHILE

Lay offs are desirable. You need a rest from any regular activity or work. Who said that "after a thousand years in heaven, a day in hell would be a pleasant change"? I'm not so sure I would want to be in hell for even a minute, but the point is well taken. Occassional lay offs from workouts will do you nothing but good. After a week or two (more if you wish) you will return to your exercising with renewed enthusiasm.

As editor of the weight-training magazine, *Muscle Mag International,* I am frequently asked by readers about training facilities in far off places. They write that they will be going on vacation in Spain, Haiti, Southern Tanzania or some other out of the way place. (I even had a query from a lady who was going to spend a week on the Isle of Elba.) Then they ask me to recommend a gym in the area.

If I can help I will, but usually I am not familiar with remote training facilities. My advice to these people who "must" train fifty-two weeks a year is: take it easy, at *least* on your vacation. On holiday you should relax in the sun, sightsee, maybe play a little tennis and swim, but forget your formal workouts. The rest will do you a world of good. And after a layoff you will be eager to return to your training routine.

If you lay off for more than a few months, be careful of your eating habits. Remember your regular training sessions burn up a considerable number of calories, and when you stop you should eat less, otherwise you may add some unwanted fat.

Generally speaking when you stop training nothing much happens except that you lose the *edge* on your muscle tone, fitness and strength. If you lay off for a period of years you will gradually return to the physical shape you were in before you took up formal exercise. If you were fat, then you may gain weight, and if you were thin, you may lose weight.

When you return to training after a layoff, even if only for a few weeks, *never* try to take up where you were prior to the layoff. Begin with lighter resistance and be content to take a week or two (more if you have been away from your workouts for an extended period) to get back to your regular regimen.

VI

HOME OR GYM TRAINING?

There are pros and cons for both training in the comfort and convenience of your home, and in joining a specialized gym.

Your main consideration in training at home is whether or not you have adequate room. What may be adequate for some people is downright cramped for others. What is really necessary is enough room to extend a barbell to arm's length above your head without touching the ceiling, and space to do lateral movements with weights. Desirable but not essential, is enough ceiling height to be able to use a jump-rope without catching it on door knobs or hitting the walls or ceiling.

Minimum equipment is a *barbell/dumbell set* and an *adjustable incline bench*. So you will need room for these plus enough space to maneuver around them without bumping into the bench or stubbing your toe on a ten pound disc. *Squat stands* are pretty essential if you are training for sports or strength.

There are literally thousands of "home gyms" set up in apartment bedrooms, kitchens, and T.V. rooms. One middle-aged lady enthusiast I know actually has an incline bench built into a walk-in closet. Her husband doesn't like to see her exercising and insists on her keeping virtually out of sight while she trains. Perhaps her efforts to be fit and trim give him a guilt complex. He could certainly use a little training himself.

Of course the "bench in the bedroom" situation is not entirely satisfactory to most because it's not particularly glamorous, and gets in the way. Far more preferable is an exercise room of your own. That is to say, a room totally devoted to your exercise sessions. That way you know exactly where you are, and you won't be in your husband's way when he's doing the dishes (hopefully?). Nor will you be performing bench presses while the family is watching its favorite T.V. show.

You may not be able to be choosy about the room you use for training, but if you have a choice, choose one that offers fresh air and natural light. A training area with windows is definitely superior to one with four blank walls, unless the room is so spacious that it makes little difference.

Assuming you have the space for a "home gym" there is another point to ponder. Unfortunately a home gym can lead to missed workouts. It's the same old story. You have a gym right there and it's not used because it is so close. You may find yourself *putting off* your workouts until later—finally after watching *just one more* T.V. program you find that you are too tired to train. This may not sound like a valid point but it happens over and over again. I have a home gym and it happened to me (I'm ashamed to admit) countless times.

On the other hand, if you are a member of a commercial gym you usually set a definite time at which to go, and once there, in the proximity of other trainers, you will probably work faster and harder and presto! You're finished and the workout's completed.

A home trainer can get "caught up" with incessant (and at your workout time, unneeded) visitors, telephone calls and unexpected domestic situations, all of which can and will interfere with your thrice weekly appointments with your barbells.

I don't mean to say or infer that home training is a waste of time. On the contrary, there will be times when the car breaks down, or the weather is so bad, that even gym workouts are impossible.

The decision is yours. But you should be aware now of the pitfalls.

The main advantages of training at a commercial gym are the wide variety of apparatus and training facilities, and the helpful atmosphere of being surrounded by other exercisers.

The last point *is* important. Being part of a gym-gang inspires quality workouts. You tend to get on with the job at hand. There is both the seen and unseen presence of competition even among your friends. You find yourself working at your exercises in a businesslike fashion. No goofing off or creeping into the den to watch the "box" between sets. In the gym it's exercise—and that's the name of the game.

Naturally, your decision to train at home or in a commercial gym relies on other factors. There may not be a gym in your vicinity. Or at least not one suitable for your requirements. Or worse, the membership fees may not be within your budget. Also you may have small children who cannot be left alone, or an invalid for whom you must be on call.

Home or commercial gym?

A weighty decision that only you can make. Think it over and decide for yourself. You and only you know the answer.

WHAT DO I HAVE TO BUY?

Assuming you opt to train at home, there is really not a great deal that you absolutely *must* acquire. But like fishing, photography, hunting or any other hobby there are many gadgets and extras that you can buy if you want to—if you have the funds. Basically though, all you *need* are:

1. A set of weights (which includes a bar and two dumbell rods, collars and sleeves).
2. An adjustable incline bench.
3. A pair of squat stands (if you choose to do regular squats).

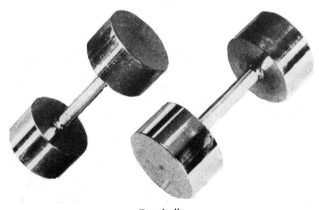

Dumbells

Most sports stores sell weights, and 110 pound sets will cost between $50–$60, depending on what it is made of and how well finished it is. Some weight sets are rather rough in finish, others are smooth, well cast and nicely painted. Chrome sets are a different kettle of fish altogether. Instead of having to pay around 60 cents a pound as you may for regular sets, you will be lucky to acquire chromed weights for anything less than $3 or $4 a pound.

The weight set you will be shown in a sports store will likely be of cast iron or vinyl. Cast iron weights last longer, gain in value (as the cost of raw iron increases) and generally are easier to handle (getting on and off the bar). They are more expensive than vinyl weights, noisier in use, and harder on carpets. Vinyl weights are filled with concrete and may "split" if they are continually dropped. Cast iron weights are virtually indestructible. I prefer cast iron, but it is a matter of individual preference.

Buying an incline bench is trickier. You need one that will support both you and the weights, have the correct dimensions and of course be sufficiently padded for comfort. At present, few stores carry acceptable weight training benches of any kind. I strongly recommend that you purchase your adjustable incline bench from one of the following companies:

Lou Ferrigno Sports Equipment, 6318 Bay Parkway, Brooklyn, N.Y. 11204.

York Barbell Company, Box 1707, York, Pa. 17405

Iron Man Industries, Box 10, Alliance, Neb. 69301.

Weider International, 21100 Erwin St., Woodland Hills, Ca. 91367.

Health Culture, Canada, Unit One, 270 Rutherford Rd. South, Brampton, Ont., Canada, L6W 3K7.

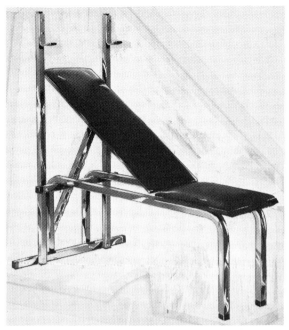

Adjustable incline bench

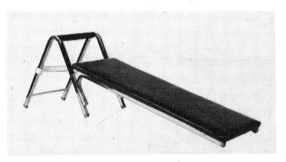

Incline board

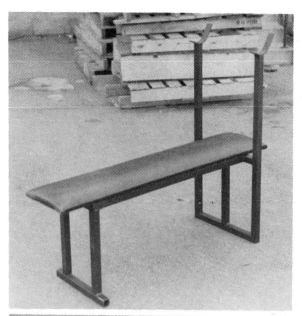

Regular flat bench

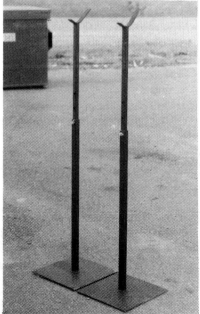

Squat stands

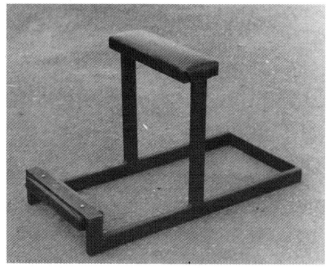

Roman chair

Each company will send you a catalog. You can buy directly from them or else they will supply a list of local stores that carry their products. The same goes for squat stands. A well made, inexpensive set of stands is not easy to find in local sports stores. The companies listed above all carry them.

There are two pieces of apparatus that could be described as "not necessary but nice to have."

The first is a Roman Chair, which enables you to perform the bent leg situp, a great waistline toner. The traditional incline board can substitute. You don't need both. And, neither are *absolutely* necessary.

Finally, somewhat of a luxury, is the thigh extension, leg curl bench. This is for ladies who don't like squatting movements. The extension bench allows you to work the front, sides and back of the thighs without doing squats. Again this apparatus is not usually found in your regular sports store but more often in "body-building stores" (which are few and far between). If in doubt look in the yellow pages under "gym equipment" or write one of the aforementioned companies.

CHOOSING A GOOD GYM

If you decide to do all your training in a commercial gym, there are a few pointers to bear in mind before you sign on the dotted line. If there is only one gym in your general area then you are pretty limited. You'll have to train there or not at all. On the other hand, most towns and cities have an abundance of training facilities, just consult your yellow pages, (look under *Gymnasiums*) and more than likely you will find yourself in a position to "choose for yourself."

Most training establishments, today, are pretty satisfactory, honest and above board. Things were not always that way. Remember, the prime concern of any commercial gym is to make money. What you should be concerned with is "do they give *value* for money?"

Don't sign a contract without first "sleeping" on it. Most big gyms (especially those which are part of a commercial gym chain) have sophisticated sales people who will try to get you to sign a one to three years contract. It may be a very worthwhile establishment, but don't get bullied into signing or joining anything you are not one hundred percent in favor of. Here are some answers you can give the sales person when he or she attempts to cajole you into signing on the dotted line, even before you know fully:

a) Whether you *really* like the place.
b) Whether you can get there *easily*.
c) Whether you have full medical *approval* from your doctor.
d) Whether you can really afford it.
e) Whether it has all the *facilities* you need.

Your curtest and most effective answer to any salesman is simply, "No". You can always soften that to "No *thank you*," (but "no" is difficult for some people to say). It takes years to learn how to say "No" with effectiveness and besides it invariably encourages a salesperson to ask you, "Don't you want to be fit?", or "Our special offer is only available today, we may not be able to offer membership at this low price again." Then you will be reminded of all the positive points again and again. You can't cut him short by interrupting because he doesn't give you time. You will be badgered until you look ready to grab the pen and sign. But don't! Instead tell the salesperson you are sure that what he says is true, but you have promised yourself never to sign any contract without sleeping on it first. Or else say that you have to consult a friend, or that you don't have any signing privileges, or that you can't write. Or that you just don't like the place. Or that orange (or whatever color the gym is) makes you sick. Or that you have to leave because you are late for a hospital appointment; your doctor suspects you may be a carrier of the new Asian plague and he wants to quarantine you before you come in contact with *too* many people. Also, you could find an easy exit by telling the salesperson that you are in fact a gym owner yourself and you were just checking on your competitors' sales approach. Remember this—when the sales person counters your negative reply with a question (this is a favorite way of drawing you back into a two-way conversation about the establishment) you are quite within your rights in saying: "Look, I don't have to explain or justify myself in *any* way. I have told you I will think about it, and if I decide to join this gym I will let you know. OK?" The salesperson may be a little taken back, but he will respect you for putting him in his place.

One last "line" to put down an over-insistent salesperson is to say that you are very "taken" by the place, but before you make any binding decisions you have to check their business and financial status through your lawyers and bankers. Because the last club you joined went out of business and you lost your enrollment fee.

How do you know whether you are looking over a good or bad gym? If there are a lot of electrical devices such as vibrator belts and roller machines, and the salesman insists that these will help you lose pounds, forget it. The main tools for bodyshaping are barbells, dumbells, running pathways, skipping or treadmill areas, benches, pulleys and sturdy exercise stations.

A thick pile carpet, soft music, chromed apparatus and freezing air conditioning don't make the best training quarters. Rather, look for simple strong apparatus and most of all an enthusiastic group of people training.

If everybody on the gym floor is sitting around talking, chances are you will be doing the same if you join. Look for a "busy" gym floor that will be contagious enough to make you train hard and progress. The clanging of barbells and dumbells on the gym floor is the right music for you. Not Frank Sinatra singing "My Way" while the gym members sit around the juice bar discussing their next door neighbors. Check the days that the gym is open. If they cater to men too you may only be able to train every other day, which might not suit your schedule.

Better to look for a commercial gym that is open to you at least six (preferably seven) days a week. I'm not suggesting you train daily, three times a week is usually suggested, but it's always nice to know that if you have to miss a workout, you can always "go in" the next day.

Incidentally, if the gym also caters to men, that is a good sign that the equipment is probably suitable. Not many gyms are "modern" enough to have men and women training together, but those that do, are usually most successful. Gold's in Santa Monica is one and probably the best gym in the world for producing results. Men and women train side by side.

Naturally, if you don't go for the idea of training alongside men then don't do it. The decision is yours.

Sometimes self consciousness enters into the decision of joining a gym. Fear of others seeing you is common. Curiously, women with the least to be self conscious about are often the most. If you are embarrassed by your present shape, remember there are bound to be others at the gym in the same condition. In fact, those who attend gyms are the people least likely to make fun of you. Whether you are a skinny 70 pound "bag of bones" or a 400 pound "sack of potatoes" you will not be laughed at. Rather, as you start to improve your condition you will become the subject of enthusiastic praise and sincere admiration.

Gym fees vary greatly. Shop around and compare. Do not buy what you are not likely to use. Beware of package memberships. Some gyms allow monthly pay-as-you-train payments, with no contracts. This of course is ideal.

VII

YOUR FIRST WORKOUT

Your first workout is important in more ways than one. Since weight training is the most concentrated form of exercise known, I can't stress too strongly that your first few workouts should be performed with very light resistance. Unless you are naturally strong, well conditioned and superbly fit right now, use *only* the bar for your first workout! Later as you gain strength you will add some discs to increase resistance.

Sets and reps

To recap, "reps" (repetitions) is used to describe the number of times you perform a particular exercise. For example, if you lift a weight up and down ten times that is known as ten repetitions.

A "set" is one *group of repetitions*. As an example if

you did ten squats that is known as *one* set of *ten* reps, (usually written 1 x 10). If you do another group (set) of squats, this is known as two sets of ten reps (written 2 x 10).

Beginners sets and reps

Beginners should do *only one set* per exercise. In two weeks this can be increased to *two sets* per exercise. In four weeks one can graduate to *three sets*. There is seldom any need to perform more than three sets of any exercise.

Repetitions are most effective in the eight to twelve range. Some women will feel they get more from fewer repetitions (six to eight) while others may prefer performing more (fifteen to twenty). For those completely in the dark about how many repetitions to do, we advise ten.

Exercise performance

When you lift a weight, the movement should always be smooth and rhythmic. There is no value in struggling with the barbell, leaning backwards to "hoist" it overhead, or bending your knees to jerk it into position. Fluid movement, exercise without strain, is what is needed. Try to raise the weight at the same speed that you lower it up-down, up-down. Keep a rhythm.

Another "must". Whenever you lift, make sure that you perform the exercise through its entire range of movement. This will mean that whenever you bend your arms during an arm, shoulder or chest exercise, make sure the arm is always straightened (locked-out) during each repetition. The same, of course, with exercises which involve the legs. Lock-out on each extension. In this way you will always be involving your muscles to their fullest. And of course, you will be ensuring total flexibility.

Breathing

Breathing during your exercise is important. Come to think of it, *breathing* is important—period, right? Try to breathe between your repetitions. Usually a gulp of air is taken just before the *hardest* part of a movement. And released just as the repetition is *completed*. Try not to hold your breath for any length of time while training. Except in a few non-strenuous movements one should breathe once with each repetition; a quick gulp of air through the mouth, exhaling through pursed lips. Unlike calisthenics, one should not breathe through the nose during weight training exercise.

Rest periods

After each set of exercises you should take a rest. Either take a brief walk around your exercise area or simply stand still. Sitting down is permissible, but not particularly recommended. In the early stages of your training rest for two minutes between sets of exercises. As you gain strength and stamina try to reduce your rest period. Aim ultimately to rest only one minute between sets. As a general guide, you should rest long enough for your breathing rate to return to normal.

Concentration

Few things help you more than concentration. Keep your mind on your exercises and results will come quickly. When you are exercising, you should watch yourself in a mirror to keep an eye on your form and control. With practice you can learn to shut out distraction. Don't carry on a running conversation while training. Keep your mind on what you are doing. In time you will be able to be in a "world of your own" during the half minute or so you devote to each set. If a bomb went off behind your back, you should hardly notice it.

When to increase the weight

The question of when to increase the weight resistance is often puzzling to beginners. The answer of course is that you add more weight when the resistance you are using feels too light. Weight training should be pleasurable. You will continually have to increase the resistance as you get stronger. But *not* to the extent of making each exercise an all-out super human effort. Train, don't strain. When you can easily do four or five more repetitions than you have planned for a particular movement, that is the time to increase the resistance. You seldom will need to add more than a couple of two and one-half pound discs at a time.

Always use barbell collars

Don't train without making sure that your weights are secure. Collars should be fastened tightly onto all barbells and dumbells. The last thing you want is a five pound disc slipping from the bar onto your big toe.

You should also make sure that the discs on either

side of the bar are equi-distant from the center. In other words, the barbell should be properly balanced, at least within an inch or so.

How long should a workout be?

Workouts vary in length from one person to another. At first, while you are getting used to performing each exercise, your workout will be longer. Maybe 30 minutes or so. Soon you will be able to cut it down to 15 minutes—maybe less. If you really "get into" weights and have a yearning to reach a peak for a beauty contest, or even a specific photo session, then you may want to add a few extra movements which inevitably will tend to increase the time of your workout. However, don't make the common mistake of thinking that more exercises, or more sets will necessarily increase the effectiveness of your training. Each person has a different tolerance to weights. What one woman will find only adequate, another will find too demanding. You must not overwork to the point that you feel overtired and drained the next day. Too much exercise is worse than none. If you overtrain you will become listless, and bored—and probably end up wanting to forget the whole thing.

The exercises (beginners)

Every workout should begin with a general warmup period. This can take the form of a two minute run, four minutes on an exercise bicycle, or a minute spent skipping or running in place. The choice is yours. But don't neglect it. Not only does a warm-up prepare your muscles for their workout, but it will also make you *feel* like training.

Exercise number one: upright rowing

Shoulders, back, arms, neck, posture.
Starting poundage: 25 pounds.

(a) Begin by holding light barbell as shown in Fig. 1. Note elbows are locked-out. Feet 12 inches apart.
(b) Raise the bar to position (Fig. 2) whereby the elbows are held high, and bar is brought almost to the chin.
(c) Lower and repeat. Keep upright throughout the exercise. Do not lean forward.

Breathing
Inhale just before bending arms. Exhale as arms are lowered across chest.

Exercise number two: hack lifts

Thighs, hips, lower back, calves.
Starting poundage: 30 pounds.

(a) Stand as shown in Fig. 3. Legs approximately 12″ apart, heels on a two inch block (or on two thick books).
(b) Slowly lower into *hacklift* position. Keep back flat, head up and keep barbell close to back of thighs.
(c) Return to original position. Do not lean too far forward.

Breathing
Inhale as you lower into the squatting position. Exhale forcefully as you straighten up.

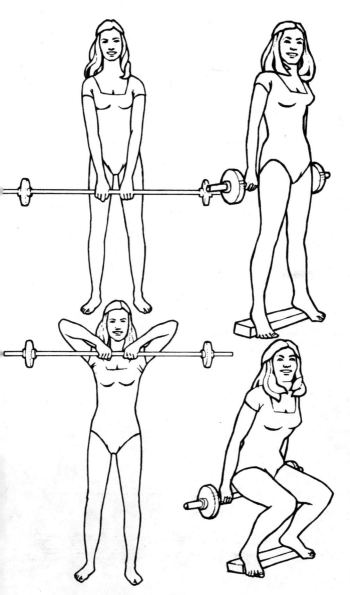

Figs. 1 and 2 Upright rowing   **Figs. 3 and 4 Hack lift**

Exercise number three: bench press

Chest, arms, shoulders.
Starting poundage: 30 pounds.

   (a) Lie on a sturdy bench with feet placed firmly on the ground.
   (b) Have a partner hand you a light barbell at arm's length as shown in Fig. 5.
   (c) Lower slowly to position (Fig. 6) and immediately return weight to arm's length, keep elbows out to the sides rather than in near the bench.

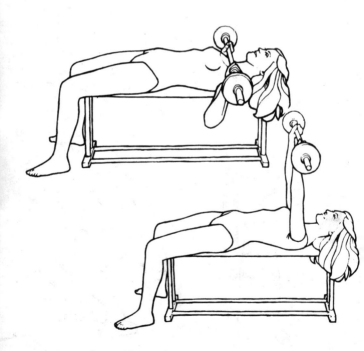

Figs. 5 and 6 Bench press

    (d) Continue this up/down movement without "bouncing" weight on the chest.

Breathing
Inhale as you lower the bar to the sternum. Breathe out as the arms straighten.

Note: Some flat benches are fitted with "rests" on which the barbell can be placed. This eliminates the need for a second person to assist in getting the barbell into the starting position.

Exercise number four: calf raise

Lower legs.
Starting poundage: 25 pounds.

    (a) Assume position shown in Fig. 7.
    (b) Be careful to maintain balance, and raise up on toes as high as possible; (Fig. 8).

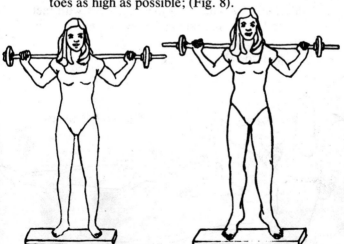

Figs. 7 and 8 Calf raise

(c) Lower and repeat. You may find it more advantageous to place toes on a two inch high wooden block (or books). This enables you to give more "stretch" to the lower leg area.

Breathing
Breathe in and out as you feel the need. One does not have to breathe once for every repetition when performing this movement.

Note: If you have difficulty in balancing you may ask a friend to steady you at first. After a week or so you should have developed the necessary balance to work alone.

Exercise number five: situps

Abdominal muscles and general midsection.
No weights required.

(a) Begin by lying on a mat or carpet with feet together as illustrated (Fig. 9).
(b) Curl body upwards until you are in the seated position shown in Fig. 10.

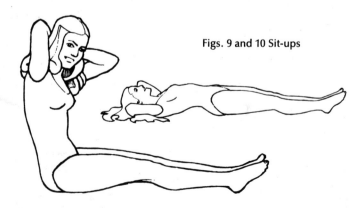

Figs. 9 and 10 Sit-ups

(c) To avoid discomfort you may place your chin on your upper chest and "round" your back as you raise up.

Breathing

Inhale just before sitting up. Breathe out as you reach the upright position (Fig. 10).

Note: You may find that you need to secure your feet under a loaded barbell (couch or bed) to avoid raising your feet as you attempt to sit up.

Exercise number six: side twists

Overall waistline and lower back.

(a) Stand up straight, feet ten inches apart, arms folded as shown in Fig. 11.
(b) Twist from side to side going as far as you can to each extremity.
(c) Try to keep hip area facing front.

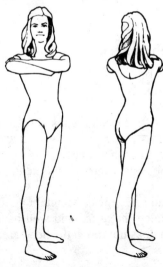

Figs. 11 and 12 Side twists

Note: This is an exercise that does not follow the normal repetition requirements. Beginners should perform at least 50 repetitions (25 each side). Work up to 200 per workout.

The foregoing weight training schedule should be performed three times weekly. Each exercise (with the exception of exercise number six) should be performed using ten repetitions for one set. Extra sets, with a maximum of three, may be added as progress is made.

After a period of six to ten weeks it may be desirable to change schedules. The following is a good alternative. You may, of course, revert back to the original schedule after a month or two. The change will help keep your enthusiasm high.

Alternative Schedule

Warm up with a few minutes running in place, jogging or skipping.

Exercise one: press behind neck

Shoulders, upper back, arms.
Starting poundage: 20 pounds.

(a) Assume position, with barbell resting across the back of shoulders, gripping the bar with a wide grip (Fig. 13). Feet 12 inches apart.
(b) Slowly "press" the weight into an overhead position (Fig. 14).
(c) Lower behind head and repeat. Maintain an upright stance and keep the arms held well back, so that the barbell does not touch the head area.

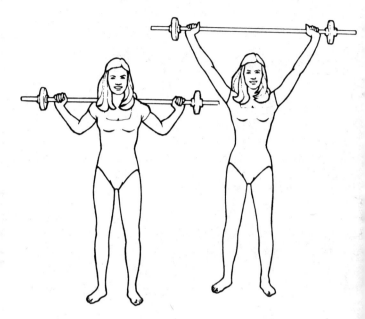

Figs. 13 and 14 Press behind neck

Breathing
Inhale before pressing the weight aloft. Exhale as arms lock-out at full extension position.

Exercise two: straddle lift squat

Thighs, hips, calves, lower back.
Starting poundage: 30 pounds.

(a) Stand as shown in Fig. 15. Feet approximately 14 inches apart.
(b) Keeping back flat and as upright as possible slowly lower into position shown in Fig. 16.
(c) Return to upright position and repeat.

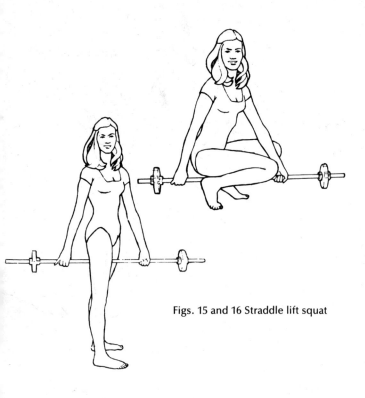

Figs. 15 and 16 Straddle lift squat

Breathing
Breathe in before lowering. Breathe out as your legs
lock out.

Note: A more popular version of this exercise, and
perhaps more comfortable, is the regular *back squat*.
This is performed in the same way, the only difference
being that the weight is held in position *behind* the
head (as though you were going to perform the press
behind the neck exercise). Lower until thighs are
parallel to the floor, and return to the upright position.
You may substitute the *back squat* for the straddle lift
squat in this routine if you wish.

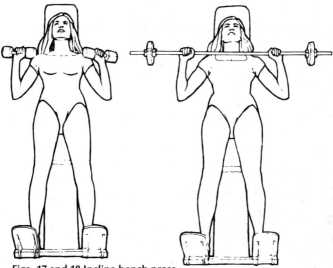

Figs. 17 and 18 Incline bench press

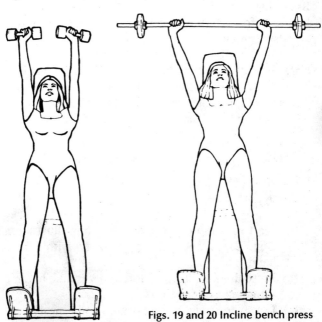

Figs. 19 and 20 Incline bench press

Exercise three: incline bench press

Upper chest, shoulders, arms.
Starting poundage: 20 pound barbell or two 10 pound
  dumbells.

(a) You may perform this exercise with dumbells or
     a single barbell. Assume position shown in
     either illustration (Figs. 19 or 20), depending on
     whether you are using a barbell or dumbell.
(b) Press weight aloft as illustrated in Figs. 17 or 18.
     The bench should be inclined at approximately
     45° angle.
(c) Lower weight to upper chest and repeat with
     rhythmic up/down motion.

Breathing
Inhale before starting the press. Breathe out as the
arms straighten.

Note: It matters little whether you use dumbells or a
barbell. Dumbells allow a little more "stretch" in the
pectoralis (upper chest) region, but may be fractionally
harder to control (balance) during the movement.

Exercise four: single arm rowing

Back, arms, shoulders.
Starting poundage: 15 pound dumbell.

(a) Start by adopting position shown in illustration
     (Fig. 21) supporting upper body with "free"
     hand.
(b) Raise dumbell keeping forearm vertical, holding
     weight close to the body (Fig. 22).
(c) Lower to straight-arm position and repeat.

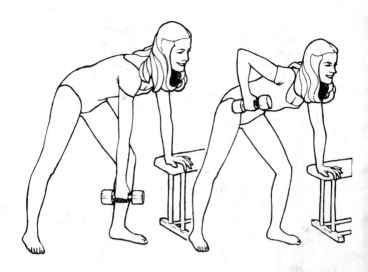

Figs. 21 and 22 Single arm rowing

(d) Change into the opposite position and holding the dumbell in the other hand, work the other side.

Breathing
Inhale once every two repetitions just before raising the weight. Exhale as it is lowered.

Exercise five: seated or incline dumbell curl

Arms, shoulders.
Starting poundage: two five pound dumbells.

(a) You may perform this exercise either seated on a standard bench (stool), or leaning back on a 45° incline bench.

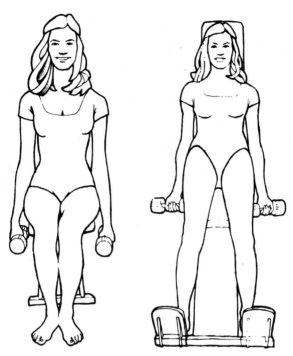

Fig. 23 Seated dumbell curl   Fig. 24 Incline dumbell curl

(b) Adopt position shown in either illustration (Fig. 23 or Fig. 24) depending on your preference.

(c) Keep the body and legs as still as possible; proceed to curl the weights into position (Figs. 25 or 26).

(d) Lower under control (don't "drop" the weights loosely) and repeat.

Breathing
Inhale while arms are straight. Exhale after curling as arms return to the hanging position.

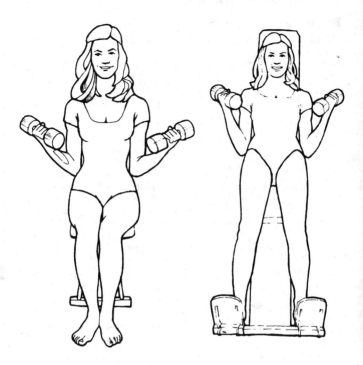

Fig. 25 Seated dumbell curl   Fig. 26 Incline dumbell curl

Exercise six: seated triceps extension

Back of arms, shoulders.
Starting poundage: two or three pound dumbell.

(a) Begin by adopting position (Fig. 27) with arm held close to the head.
(b) Feet may be together or apart depending on personal preference.
(c) By moving *only* the forearm, extend the weight to position shown in illustration (Fig. 28).
(d) Lower slowly behind neck and repeat.

Breathing

Breathe in before starting the movement. Exhale as arm straightens.

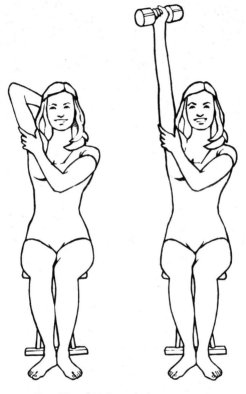

Figs. 27 and 28 Seated triceps extension

Exercise seven: side twists

Overall waist and lower back.
Starting poundage: 25 pounds.

(a) Start with bar across the back of your shoulders as shown in illustration (Fig. 29).
(b) Slowly twist into position (Fig. 30) and then return to original front position.
(c) Twist to the other side, return and repeat.

Breathing
Inhale and exhale when you find it most comfortable.

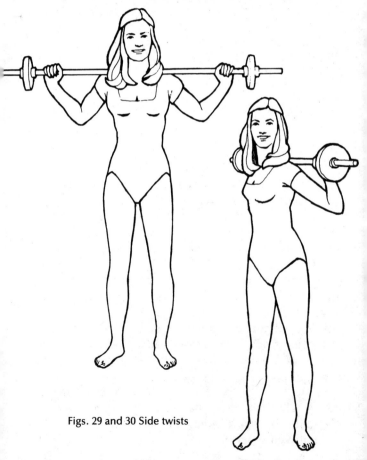

Figs. 29 and 30 Side twists

VIII

WHY PUMPING IRON IS BEST

Charles Gaines thought of and popularized through his best selling book, the now well-established name, *Pumping Iron*. This is just another name for "weight training". It caught on with the general public, and even somewhat reluctantly, with the hard core body-builders as well.

Whatever name you choose to use, be sure of one thing: it is the best darned way of "making yourself over" that has yet been devised. Yes, to date, the use of free weights in training is still superior to all the gadgets, machinery, devices and contraptions that have flooded the exercise market in the last decade or so.

True, there has been some ground gained by makers of single and multi-stationed apparatus like the Nautilus, but apart from a few units, pumping iron has still proven superior.

Nautilus

The Nautilus apparatus is not just one machine. It is a name given to a whole line of complicated machinery designed for overall body conditioning, strengthening and developing. There are many Nautilus centers throughout North America where one can train almost exclusively on these huge machines. Each unit has its specific use. There is a chest machine, an arm machine, a leg and hip machine, and so on. The idea of buying a complete Nautilus line for a home gym is extravagant. The cost would run into tens of thousands and one would require at least five hundred square feet in which to park them.

Nautilus is the brain child of entrepreneur Arthur Jones of Orlando, Florida. Jones himself is a man of controversial and original ideas on almost any subject.

He has a dozen alligators running around his Florida ranch, and claims that they respect him. There must be something to it since he's still alive.

Nautilus machines are used extensively in gyms by football players, athletes and fitness enthusiasts. They do work. Bodybuilders at one time migrated *en masse* away from standard barbells and dumbells to train exclusively with the Nautilus units, but time has shown that free weights have won the day. Most are back with their barbells and dumbells and only use Nautilus for one or two exercises, if at all. However, Arthur Jones' machinery is improving all the time and he may still end up with *the* perfect apparatus.

Universal machines

Like Nautilus, Universal exercise apparatus was also designed to take the place of free weights. Many

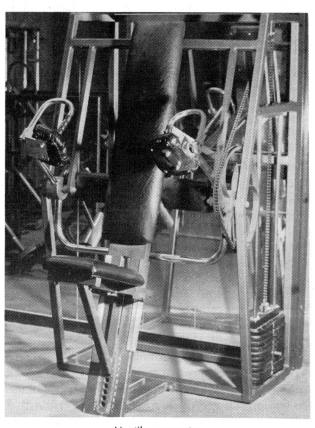

Nautilus apparatus

schools, colleges and YMCA's have installed these chromed units. Like Nautilus, they work well for most, but they do not offer the enormous variety of movements that weights do. Some of the attachments and accessories are not sturdy enough for everyone to use. Also the resistances claimed on the apparatus don't match up with similar poundages marked on weights. In other words, although you may think you are lifting 50 pounds or whatever with the Universal machine, you would not be able to perform a similar number of repetitions with a barbell. Many a youngster has been delighted to "bench press" 100 pounds on a Universal machine only to find that he couldn't budge a standard barbell, legitimately loaded with the same weight.

Doug Hepburn machine

This is an apparatus mainly for home training. The machine simulates just about any barbell and dumbell exercise, and in fact there are some exercises one can do with the Hepburn machine that cannot be done with weights.

The greatest advantage of the Hepburn exercise apparatus is the fact that resistance can be dialed instantly. In other words if you want to perform a squat exercise you can change the dial to give a resistance of 60 lbs. or so, and then within a second you can nudge the dial to give you *half* the resistance or double it; or whatever you wish. The resistance goes up to about 200 pounds, which is more than adequate for most people's needs. The Doug Hepburn machine is ideal for the whole family to use, is completely portable, and can be stored almost anywhere.

Bullworker for women

The Bullworker apparatus has enjoyed world wide sales in the millions throughout Britain, Canada, U.S.A., Australia, and Germany (where it was invented).

It is now being advertised as a figure aid for women. Looking at the Bullworker apparatus objectively one can understand that it is a useful unit for building the upper chest muscles (pectoralis); however, it's limitations are very obvious when it comes to functional leg work. In fact, because most muscles cannot be worked through their entire range of movement, it is safe to surmise that Bullworker is not an ideal exercise apparatus for the overall body, development, conditioning or slimming.

Marcy 8 Station Master gym

This is a compact multi-purpose exercise apparatus not dissimilar to the Universal setup in principle. Although these units look pleasant, and their high gloss finish can only be considered attractive, they lack the feel of free weights and their versatility. The Marcy 8 Station unit does have a cable attachment that can be used to work the important outer thigh area, but it has pronounced limitations. For example, the machine doesn't afford a variety of "grip" positions on the bar. When working with a barbell, hand position can be altered to very close, very wide, or a score of other variations. With the Marcy apparatus you can grip one position only. Thus the apparatus is not ideal for very tall or very short people.

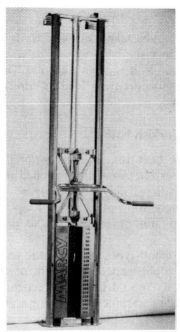
Marcy machine

Vibrator belts

Electrical gadgets which cause a wide belt to vibrate against the flesh serve no purpose other than to massage the area in which they are being used. They do not reduce fat, nor lose pounds.

Plastic suits, wraps, sauna shorts and rubberized belts

These gadgets lock in air and heat up the body. Although they may induce sweating they do not help in the loss of fat. Because water content of the body is reduced, there may be some temporary weight loss.

But as soon as you take a drink of water that weight will return, since the body always balances its liquid content as soon as it is given a chance. The body will even absorb moisture from food to bring the balance back to normal.

Sauna and Turkish baths

The intense heat from a Sauna is not always good. Like the rubberized garments mentioned above, a very hot room or bath will only temporarily induce sweating and accordingly will not either firm up the muscle, induce loss of fat nor provide any other proven physical benefit.

There are many types of apparatus and scores of gadgets and sophisticated equipment on the market. Each makes its special claim for recognition. These vary from pulley machines and rowing units to twister wheels and door knob body-shapers. As yet there are no ideal exercisers on the market—and more relevant to this book, none that can work the complete body as effectively as progressive resistance training using free weights, pumping iron.

SPOT REDUCING

The Truth

There has been a lot of talk about *spot reducing*. The term simply means "losing weight in specific areas"— for example, many women have the problem of too much weight (or flab) on the upper thighs and seat area. They want to lose weight there but not necessarily anywhere else. You've heard the old lament: "I have to lose weight off my hips, but I hate doing it because my bust shrinks to nothing."

In order to "spot reduce" certain body parts, man has come up with scores of novel ideas which range from tightly bandaging the area with special wraps, exercising the part exclusively, wearing rubberized garments, using electrical vibrator belts, pummeling with hands or motor driven units, applying various liniments and oils, massaging the individual areas, and even using electrodes to pass mild electrical currents through the problem area. All these *spot reducing* methods have three things in common:

1. They are novel and are being used all over North America and Europe.
2. They are making money for those who sell and promote them.
3. They don't work.

That's right. Spot reducing is not a workable concept. In my job as editor in chief of my own publishing company, Health Culture, Ont. Canada, I come into contact with scores of women who ask about spot reduction. A typical conversation starts with, "Mr. Kennedy, what can I do for my hips?" Or, "I need to lose weight from my tummy; what is the best exercise, situps?" This latter question is both asked and answered by the questioner. She *expects* me to reply something to the effect, "Yep! Do two sets of 25 situps every night and your tummy will vanish within a couple of weeks."

All the more surprise when I tell them that situps will do nothing for their fat tummies—NOTHING! The only thing that situps or any other direct tummy exercise will do is to firm up the actual muscle tissue *underneath* the fat. You will still be flabby, soft and obese. Here's a true story to prove my point.

When I was attending a physical education seminar at Loughborough Training College in England, I was present at a gymnasium where a fellow in his early twenties was training to break the world situps record. He later established the grand total of 7,504 which was witnessed by the staff of the Guinness Book of Records. His "training" at the time I witnessed his workouts involved performing between 2,200 and 2,500 situps each evening, six nights a week. Now here's the amazing fact. Despite having worked at his situps for 11 months and averaging around 14,000 situps weekly this fellow was—FAT!

That did it for me. I became a believer or disbeliever as the case may be. Situps are good. They firm up the underlying tissue; they help keep your internal organs toned and healthy. But they *will not rid your midsection of fat!* Think of it—If over 2,000 situps a night couldn't give this person a slim, fat-free waistline, then how on earth could a couple of sets of 20 do it for you?

Remember this: Whatever exercise you do, it will only affect your fat to the extent of the number of calories you burn up in the effort. And that fat will come off all over your body. It will not just vanish from the area worked by a particular exercise. Nor is formal exercise a great burner of calories. You have to do some pretty exhausting (or lengthy) exercises to make a significant reduction in fat.

Now wait a minute! I'm not knocking formal exercise. It generates energy, firmer, more shapely muscles, health, fitness, and a happier, more relaxed state of mind. But exercise will not *spot reduce* fat.

If you feel you have a problem "fat" area then you are probably carrying some fat all over your body—All superfluous fat is undesirable and it is removed via the application of D-I-E-T. Fewer calories. You cannot take a little fat off here and there. You lose fat all over your body in direct proportion to the reduced number of calories you take in. Your *workout* however, gives you the desirable muscular shape that becomes visible when you lose the fat. Exercise also increases the number of calories your body uses.

POSTURE

Good posture is achieved when the different segments of the body are balanced vertically on each other. When we walk, run or engage in varied activities this alignment changes. In walking for example, the upper body tends to lean or "fall" forward as we advance.

The word posture indicates the manner in which we carry the body when standing, sitting or walking. It is an ever varying pattern of stance. One changes posture every time one changes activity. This constant change becomes "second nature" to us. We get into the habit of either sitting correctly or lazily. The same with other activities. It's easy to sag, and this is where the trouble begins. Sagging can become a habit, and habits can "grow" on you. In this case—literally. If you practice bad posture long enough it will become habitual. The same of course, with good posture. Practice it and it can become you.

In spite of the fact that an upright stance is man's natural position, most people droop and become round shouldered. To avoid this "old man's stoop" make a constant effort to "correct" your posture throughout the day.

Correct posture is really the most *relaxing* posture. Curiously enough, those who think they are relaxing by slouching are really causing added fatigue to set in. Watch any sidewalk. Visit any schoolroom, audience, or football crowd. Almost everyone is slouching, which is usually an indication of physical weakness. Bad posture can contribute to illness. Lungs can be cramped; stomach, liver, and other abdominal organs can be crowded and dislodged.

Good posture is an aesthetic and a health plus. The woman who stands well—upright and proud—holds within her a beauty asset. And good posture aids verbal expression. In his book *"Exercise,"* Dr. Herbert M. Shelton states: "Upon the upright attitude depends the usefulness of the senses, complete respiration, the ability to talk, speak or read with correct tone of force and the most efficient use of the body. Erect carriage is exceedingly important to the health and vigor as well as the best appearance of man and woman."

There is no doubt that to secure the best results in function and appearance of *your* body, all of your structures must be properly aligned. Poor posture can result in stress and strain which may cause discomfort and pain.

Lordosis

The abnormal forward tilting of the pelvis is known as lordosis. This condition contributes to general abdominal malfunctions.

Kyphosis

Kyphosis results when the upper back is overly rounded. Combined, as it often is, with lordosis, it is called kyphlordosis.

Side Balance

Disturbed *lateral* balance of the spinal column gives unequal shoulder height (one is lower than the other).

This can result from one leg being shorter than the other, or from a tilted pelvis, but more often than not it results from poor "control" habits.

It is true that sometimes postural defects are inherited, such as a shorter leg or some structural fault in the spine or pelvis, but most irregularities are caused by poor habits such as sitting with one leg under the other (which causes spinal curvature) or slouching at the meal table (which causes abdominal deterioration and curved upper back).

There are certain postural malfunctions that are beyond immediate control, but most are preventable and remediable. Most can be corrected by postural awareness and by regular practice of correctional exercises. Here are a few specific corrective exercises.

Round Shoulders

Sit with hands clasped behind your head, keeping your back and head in a straight line. With hands behind your head, bring elbows as far back as possible, tightening the upper back muscles to their limit. Do this exercise every day for one set of ten repetitions.

Uneven Shoulders

Hold a dumbell (about ten to twenty pounds) in the hand of the shoulder which is low. Simply shrug that shoulder, keeping the arm straight. One set of fifteen repetitions.

Drooping Head

Sit upright in a chair, with your chin touching your upper chest. Clasp hands behind head and raise head while resisting strongly with your hands. One set of fifteen repetitions.

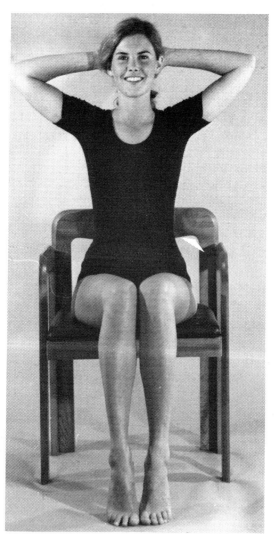

Nancy Sharp, of Toronto, Canada, shows the correct position for the seated postural exercises.

Few exercises in themselves will correct poor posture. Sports or athletic pursuits will help slightly. Some sports even contribute to severe postural *defects*. Judo and figure skating abet lower back "hollowness." Cycling and boxing help to "round" upper backs.

However, to be fair, most sports strengthen the overall skeletal muscles. Weight training does it better, because *all* the muscles are involved.

Remember this—postural improvement will result from overall strengthening exercises *plus* constant attention to *correcting* your stance whenever you catch yourself sagging or drooping.

IX

CORRECT NUTRITION

Literally billions of words have been written on nutrition; each new book more complicated than the last. We humans read unceasingly on how best to feed ourselves, yet the average jack rabbit does the job *instinctively,* and better.

Although we do what our countries ask of us by paying taxes, obeying the law, filing countless government forms, and paying into employment and pension funds which may never benefit us, we have to accept the fact that the government has let us down in the critical area that is supposed to keep us alive and kicking—food!

Magazines such as *Here's Health, Strength and Health,* and *Prevention* have questioned the danger of insecticides, food coloring, flavorings, hormones, sweeteners and food additives for years. If the government listened, they certainly didn't act. Rather they labeled the dissenters as "faddists." Now, almost daily we learn that many of these "chemicals" are carcinogenic. That's right.

Thousands of lives will be shortened because we believed that *no* government would ever allow harmful or carcinogenic agents into foods we eat daily. And yet it *has* happened. We now know that food we ate, ten, twenty, or thirty years ago may cause cancer. How many women the world over trusted the "tested" drug thalidomide, yet gave birth to deformed children? What about the cancer-causing food dyes that governments have allowed us to ingest without warning. Can you imagine contracting a *fatal* disease because a food company wanted their meat, sauce, or fruit, to *look* brighter than nature colored it? Did you want redder meat, pinker cherries, yellower pears or greener cabbage?

And what about hormones? Profits are increased if you feed your cattle anabolic steroids (hormones) but what they forget to tell us is that we too will increase our hormone level, another cancer risk.

One night Johnny Carson joked: "Today was a very remarkable day. No one discovered a new cause of cancer." The audience laughed. But Johnny was wrong. That very same day the New York Times carried a feature asserting that hamburger was the newest cause of cancer!

Have you ever had a hot dog headache? You may have had one without knowing it was caused by the hot dog. The villain is an additive, sodium nitrate typically found in ham, bacon, luncheon meats and sausage.

So what does one do? How can one live if everything we eat and drink is poisonous? As I see it, you have three choices. You can (1) eat a total junk diet—colas, hot dogs, sugar-based pastries and drinks, candies, synthetic cookies—in fact anything that takes your fancy. Or you can (2) limit junk foods to "eating out," while sticking to wholesome natural foods the rest of the time. Your third choice is to insist on 100% unadulterated foods grown in totally natural soil—fresh meats and fish that are unpolluted; whole grain cereal that has not been made spongy to seem fresher, or bleached to look whiter, or dipped in saccharin to taste sweeter.

I believe a diet of junk foods will definitely hurt you in the long run.

It is fairly easy to take the middle path and be selective. Buy fresh fruits, lean meats, fish and vegetables. There are government regulations now that at least partly protect us from the really heavy killers, but make no mistake about it, we are not, and never have been, told all the truth.

Your third alternative, eating only health foods, sounds good in theory. But actually getting food that is guaranteed unadulterated is very difficult. In fact, it is impossible for millions of families to find daily access to absolutely pure food.

So what do I recommend? Follow the dictates of Dr. Michael Walczak, the most knowledgeable man I know on nutrition. In his book, *Nutrition and Well Being* (Mojave Books) Walczak asks you to bear in mind three points about nutrition.

1. Select foods which are basically healthy.
2. *Your food intake is the "key" to your bodyshaping progress.* Training alone will not shape your body. It must be coupled with correct nutrition.
3. Although a balanced diet is important, it is the *amount* of your general food intake (overall calories) coupled with your training which will determine whether you gain or lose. A balanced

diet consists of a variety of fresh fruits, fresh vegetables, salads, meat, fish, fowl, eggs, cheeses and whole grain or cereal products.

The foods that you should stay clear of for 99% of your meals are: Canned fruits in syrup or sugar, colas, bleached white bread, salt (there's natural salt in fruits and vegetables), the general run of cakes, chocolate, candy bars, commercial cereals (which are mainly sugar), pastas, spaghetti, strong coffee, charcoal steaks, hot dogs, synthetic creams (often spelled kreme, creem, creme, kream, or kreem). The latter names are used to protect the manufacturer from false claims but still be associated with the real thing. Stay away from T.V. dinners, white flour products, gooey, sweet smelling cookies, buns, pretzels, potato chips and pastries.

Keep sugar out of the house. There is more than enough in fruits and vegetables. Honey is a good substitute if you must have an extra sweetener.

What about beer and other alcohol? Not recommended, but an occasional drink, especially with a meal, is acceptable.

Someone once said, "I have never known a totally healthy person who was consumed by the idea of being healthy." If I were to suggest how you should eat, I would say *don't be a fanatic. Try your best to eat good, wholesome natural foods whenever possible. But, if you're out on a date, or with friends or family, then by all means have a couple of drinks, slurp up that special ice cream or soda pop, relish that gooey pastry covered with artificial gunk. But keep this type of eating in hand.* Remember—99% of your eating should be the good stuff—natural yogurt, not sugary substitutes, pure juices instead of sweetened "fruit" drinks (which may contain no fruit at all) whole wheat bread instead of spongy, bleached white bread. Lean meats as opposed to spicey, dressed up, artificially colored substitutes—and so on.

To function efficiently, your body needs a combination of carbohydrates, fats, vitamins, minerals and water. No one food contains everything you need, although milk comes pretty near it. Some foods are good for one element yet only contain minimal amounts of the others. Let's take a look at these different elements.

Protein

Protein is essential for the building and repairing of the body cells. It is needed even when you are on the most rigid diet to *lose* weight, not just when you're trying to build up.

During digestion protein is broken down into eight essential acids. The body cannot manufacture them, so you must ingest them on a regular basis.

A food has high nutritional value when it contains a large quantity of amino acids.

The main protein foods are meat, fish, eggs, cheese, milk and milk products, soya beans, poultry, peas, nuts, grains and cereals.

Carbohydrates

Carbohydrates consist of sugars and starches. They are the body's principle source of energy. (If your carbohydrates are low your body may utilize protein for energy.) As you know, the body stores excess carbohydrates as "fat."

Carbohydrate sources include potatoes, cereals, bread, cakes, crackers, spaghetti (and other pasta), rice, bananas, lima beans, corn, dried fruits, syrups, jellies, jams, honey, sugar, candy, and soft drinks.

Fats

Fats are used primarily as an energy source, but they are also instrumental in protecting the various internal organs. They help to regulate body temperature and some supply large quantities of needed vitamins.

Fat sources are butter, margarine, cream, fatty meats, most cheeses, salad dressing, mayonnaise, egg yolks, nuts, fried foods, chocolate, rich desserts, peanut butter and shortenings.

Minerals

The bones and teeth contain large amounts of the minerals calcium and potassium. However, other minerals are required to balance the body processes. Nerves, muscles and organs require body fluids containing such minerals as sodium, potassium and calcium.

The most important minerals are: calcium (for teeth and bones); copper (for blood vessel normality); iodine (for energy regulation); iron (for prevention of anemia); magnesium (for building bones); phosphorus (for regulating metabolism); potassium (for healthy nerves and muscles); sodium (for absorption of glucose, and balancing the body acid-base); zinc (for normal growth and development).

Vitamins

Vitamins are needed so that food can be utilized and the body function properly.

Vitamins A, D, E, and K (fat soluble) are not needed daily. However, vitamins C and B (water soluble) *are* required daily. Excess is excreted in the urine.

Deficiencies show up rapidly. Here are some of the vitamins and a few of their uses.

Vitamin A for healthy bones, skin, teeth, resistance to infection, and good vision. It is found in eggs, cheese, liver, tomatoes, butter, milk and milk products and margarine.

Vitamin B_1 (Thiamine) for a healthy nervous system. It is found in pork, organic meats such as liver, kidney, heart, and in whole grain breads, cereals, peas, nuts, beans and eggs.

Vitamin B_2 (Riboflavin) helps in the use of protein, fats and carbohydrates for energy and tissue building. It promotes healthy skin, particularly around the mouth, nose and eyes. It is found in organ meats, liver sausage, milk, cheese, eggs, whole grain bread, dried beans, and leafy green vegetables.

Niacin promotes a healthy nervous system and skin, aids normal digestion, helps cells use oxygen to release energy. It is found in liver, meats, fish, whole grain breads, dried peas and beans, peanut butter and nuts.

Vitamin B_6 (Pyridoxine) aids in protein utilization and prevention of certain types of anemia. It is also helpful in maintaining normal growth. It is found in liver, kidneys, butter, meats, as well as in fish, cereal, soy beans, tomatoes, peanuts and corn.

Pantothenic Acid helps in the breakdown of fats, proteins and carbohydrates for energy. It is found in organ meats, egg yolk, meats, fish, soy beans, peanuts, broccoli, cauliflower, potatoes, peas, cabbage, and whole grain products.

Folic Acid promotes the development of red blood cells, and the normal metabolism of carbohydrates, proteins and fats. It is found in organ meats, asparagus, turnips, spinach, kale, broccoli, corn, cabbage, lettuce, potatoes, and nuts.

Vitamin B_{12} produces red blood cells in bone marrow, and builds new proteins. It helps the normal functioning of nervous tissue. It is found in liver, kidneys, lean meats, fish, hard cheeses and milk.

Vitamin C (Ascorbic Acid) helps "cement" cells together. It produces healthy teeth, gums, and blood vessels; and improves iron absorption. It hastens the healing of wounds and resistance to infections. It also aids in the synthesis of hormones that regulate body functions. It is found in citrus fruits (grapefruit, oranges, lemons), strawberries, cantaloupes, raw vegetables (especially green peppers), cauliflower, broccoli, kale, tomatoes, potatoes, cabbage and brussels sprouts.

Vitamin D promotes healthy bones and teeth and helps the body absorb calcium and phosphorus. Found in liver, egg yolk, foods fortified with Vitamin D such as Vitamin D Milk. It is produced by exposure to direct sunlight.

Vitamin E protects red blood cells and retards destruction of Vitamin A and C. It is found in wheat germ oil, rice, leafy vegetables, nuts, margarine and legumes.

Vitamin K permits blood clotting. It is found in spinach, kale, cabbage, cauliflower and pork liver.

I said earlier that food intake (calories) is the key to bodybuilding success. The more you ingest, the heavier you'll be. The fewer calories you ingest, the lighter you'll be. You can choose your weight.

Calorie control is the only way

Few people are happy with the way they look. Are you a naturally "skinny" person? You probably have a "high" metabolism. Are you overweight? Obese? Skinny or fat, with the help of this program you can change for the better. You can remake yourself!

Let's forget about the dumbells and barbells for a minute, and talk DIET CHANGE.

Here are the thermodynamic facts that will help you normalize your weight.

When a body takes in as many calories as it burns up (a calorie is a unit of heat energy) this is known as THERMODYNAMIC BALANCE. ("Thermo" means heat; "dynamic" refers to movement.)

If you ingest fewer calories you will lose weight; more, and you will gain.

One way of simplifying thermodynamics is to look at it like a bank account. You start with a given amount of money in the bank (fat on your body). Eating corresponds to making deposits. Exercise (walking, breathing, running) can be regarded as writing a check. If your deposits equal your withdrawals, your balance (weight) will stay the same. Burn more calories than you consume and your body will start losing weight. If you eliminate just one pat of butter a day, you won't deposit some 3,780 calories each month! This represents one pound of fat "burned off"—12 pounds a year. Eliminate two pats of butter a day and you'll lose about half a pound a week.

A word of caution: any diet should be balanced nutritionally. To simply choose a menu of low calorie foods is *not* satisfactory. Foods should never be evaluated strictly on their calorie count.

Opinions vary as to exactly how much, and what kind of foods we require for a balanced eating program. But generally speaking, one should select foods from each of the five main groups.

1. *Milk group*—Milk, cheese, ice cream
2. *Meat group*—Beef, veal, lamb, pork, poultry, eggs, fish
3. *Vegetable/fruit group*—(the fresher the better)

4. *Bread/grain group*—(whole wheat, enriched or restored)
5. Fats/oil group—Butter, margarine (usually only a small amount of these)

It may be advisable to supplement your diet with a multi-vitamin-mineral tablet each day. More about that later.

Getting Back to Calories

As a quick guide you can say that a "cut" of 500 calories per day will take off one pound per week, 50 pounds in a year! A daily cut of 1000 calories will leave you two pounds lighter every week, and so on. The same arithmetic applies if you want to gain.

You should know how many calories you are presently consuming. Count them up as you go through your usual day. Don't miss any. Remember, if you have a quick snack, or a piece of chocolate and don't record it on your daily calorie total, you are cheating no one but yourself. *It is an accepted opinion that a person leading a moderately active life needs 15 calories per pound of body weight, every day.*

So, look at the weight/height charts along with this program and find out how much you should weigh. (These charts can never be perfect, but they do give an *indication*.)

Multiply your desired weight by 15 and the answer is the number of calories you need to ingest daily to maintain that weight.

As an example, if you want to weigh 150 pounds you should be eating 2,250 calories a day just to keep at that weight.

We suggest that you do not try to alter your weight by more than 1 or 2 lbs. per week (100 lbs. per year).

This is considered a safe rate at which to lose weight. You should not normally eat less than 1000–1200 calories a day, unless you do so under a doctor's supervision.

Your normal weight

Height/weight tables are really only a rough guide. The best way to tell if you are overweight is to take a skinfold test at the triceps of the arm, as this determines whether your weight is muscle or fat. Remember the test? Simply pinch some of your skin between your thumb and forefinger. If your pinched skin is more than half an inch, this indicates that you are carrying too much fat.

Your main guide should be the triceps skinfold test *and* your bedroom mirror. However, we are including a much used height/weight table for both sexes so that you may see how you presently compare.

Metabolism

Metabolism is the rate at which your body burns fuel. Regular activity, combined with youth, often leads to a high metabolism. We all know young people who seem to gorge themselves and never gain a pound. But basal metabolism tends to slow down as the years pass by. When you eat, your metabolic rate increases. Curiously, the greatest increase in metabolic activity occurs when we eat high protein foods. In fact, the mere act of eating protein raises metabolism 30 percent above basal metabolic rate (B.M.R.) while fat raises it four percent and carbohydrates six percent. In short, the body works harder to metabolize protein than other food substances.

HEIGHT/WEIGHT TABLE (FEMALE)

HEIGHT**		SMALL FRAME		MEDIUM FRAME		LARGE FRAME	
In.	Cm.	Lb.	Kg.	Lb.	Kg.	Lb.	Kg.
6'0"	182.9	138-147	62.6-67.0	144-159	65.3-72.1	153-173	69.4-78.5
5'11"	180.3	134-144	60.8-65.3	140-155	63.5-70.3	149-168	67.6-76.2
5'10"	177.8	130-140	59.0-63.5	136-151	61.7-68.5	145-163	65.8-74.0
5'9"	175.3	126-135	57.2-61.2	132-147	59.9-66.7	141-158	64.0-71.7
5'8"	172.7	121-131	54.9-59.4	128-143	58.1-64.9	137-154	62.1-69.9
5'7"	170.2	118-127	53.5-57.6	124-139	56.2-63.1	133-150	60.3-68.1
5'6"	167.6	114-123	51.7-55.8	120-135	54.4-61.2	129-146	58.5-66.2
5'5"	165.1	111-119	50.3-54.0	116-130	52.6-59.0	125-142	56.7-64.4
5'4"	162.6	108-116	49.0-52.6	113-126	51.3-57.2	121-138	54.9-62.6
5'3"	160.0	105-113	47.6-51.3	110-122	49.9-55.3	118-134	53.5-60.8
5'2"	157.5	102-110	46.3-49.9	107-120	48.5-54.2	115-131	52.2-59.4
5'1"	154.9	99-107	44.9-48.5	104-116	47.2-52.6	112-128	50.8-58.1
5'0"	152.4	96-104	45.3-47.2	101-113	45.8-51.3	109-125	49.4-56.7
4'11"	149.8	94-101	42.6-45.8	98-110	44.4-49.9	106-122	48.1-55.3
4'10"	147.3	98	41.7-44.4	96-107	43.5-48.5	104-119	47.2-54.0

* For women between 18 and 25, subtract 1 pound for each year under 25.
**With shoes with 2 inch heels

ACTIVITY AND CALORIC REQUIREMENTS

WEIGHT	INACTIVE (Does nothing actively) Multiply your weight by 12.	MILDLY ACTIVE (Rides to work, sits at work) Multiply your weight by 14.	MEDIUM ACTIVE (Teacher, mother of small children) Multiply your weight by 16.	ACTIVE (On the move most of the time) Multiply your weight by 18.	VERY ACTIVE (Physical worker plus extra exercise) Multiply your weight by 20.
94	1140	1330	1520	1710	1900
97	1176	1372	1568	1764	1960
100	1212	1414	1616	1818	2020
104	1260	1470	1680	1890	2100
109	1320	1540	1760	1980	2200
115	1380	1615	1840	2070	2300
121	1414	1680	1920	2160	2400
124	1500	1750	2000	2250	2500
129	1560	1820	2080	2340	2600
135	1620	1890	2160	2430	2700
141	1680	1960	2240	2520	2800
146	1740	2030	2320	2610	2900
150	1800	2100	2400	2700	3000
154	1860	2170	2480	2790	3100
160	1920	2240	2560	2880	3200
164	1980	2310	2640	2970	3300
174	2100	2450	2800	3150	3500
184	2220	2590	2960	3330	3700
194	2340	2730	3120	3510	3900
200	2400	2800	3200	3600	4000
209	2520	2940	3360	3780	4200
221	2640	3080	3520	3960	4400

Faulty Nutrition

"Faulty nutrition" can be basically described as a diet which does not contain the proper ingredients, and/or the number of calories you need. Faulty nutrition is common. It is typified by diets that are loaded with carbohydrates, sugars, starches and fats. If you eat more sugars and starches than your body can immediately utilize, some is converted to a starch known as glycogen, which can be quickly reconverted to glucose when your body needs energy. However, most of the excess carbohydrates you eat are converted directly to fat.

IN DIETING TO LOSE WEIGHT, EAT A LARGE PROPORTION OF PROTEIN, NO MORE THAN 30 PERCENT FAT (MOSTLY UNSATURATED), AND A MINIMUM AMOUNT OF CARBOHYDRATES AND SUGAR. PROTEIN IS THE MOST IMPORTANT FOOD CATEGORY AND THE MOST INEFFICIENTLY DIGESTED AND ABSORBED BY THE BODY. FATS ARE NECESSARY, BUT THE REGULAR EATING OF SATURATED FATS MAY BE DANGEROUS TO THE HEART AND BLOOD VESSELS. ONLY A SMALL AMOUNT OF CARBOHYDRATES IS REQUIRED.

Women who want to gain weight should follow the proportion of ingredients advocated for weight loss, but eat more fruits and vegetables. Basically, just increase your daily calorie intake.

It is difficult to say exactly how many calories you should be taking in every day because of individual body chemistry and inherited traits. However, the table below should be helpful. Although your workouts will burn up calories, they should not be looked upon as a means of losing weight. Activities like distance running, stair climbing and squash are among the heavy calorie burners. Weight training is a means of toning, building, and shaping the body. You should rely *principally* on your diet to alter weight. A healthy nutritional program should include daily:

1. Milk or milk products (unless of course, you're allergic to milk).
2. A high protein ingredient with every meal (meat, fish, poultry, eggs, cheese, nuts).
3. Vegetables high in vitamin A (at least 4 times a week).
4. Citrus fruits (Vitamin C).
5. Whole grain breads (enriched breads/cereals).
6. Vegetable oils high in polyunsatured fat.

Eggs are not recommended as a daily requirement (3–4 eggs a week are plenty; more *may* be harmful). Children may have up to 7 a week. Poached or boiled eggs are best, but add variety to your meals by eating an egg salad sandwich or a tasty omelette now and then. Egg whites are not restricted at all since they contain no fat.

It could be said that virtually everyone needs milk every day. Milk is our best source of calcium and in order to maintain strong bones and teeth we need calcium daily.

Children can drink up to a pint of milk a day, but adults should make sure that the milk they drink is fat reduced. In other words, skim off the cream or use a fat free milk powder. You may substitute a low fat yogurt for the low-fat milk if it isn't available.

Cottage cheese or other low-fat cheeses are highly recommended. Try to stay away from the cream processed cheeses (Camembert, cheddar or Swiss cheese). They are all high in fat.

Peanut butter has enjoyed enormous popularity in North America mainly for its taste (children love it). It is an excellent food, with a high content of vegetable protein, B vitamins and unsaturated fat. It is a great sandwich spread.

Sample Diets

The following sample diets help you formulate your own eating pattern. Bear in mind what I mentioned earlier about thermodynamic balance. Ingest more calories than you need for body maintenance and you will gain weight. Eat less and you will lose.

1000 Calories

Breakfast
½ grapefruit
1 boiled egg
1 slice whole wheat bread
coffee or tea with milk (no sugar)

Mid morning
yogurt (made from partially skimmed milk, plain)

Lunch
1 cup V-8 juice
chicken salad (1 cup diced cooked chicken, with celery and 1 tbsp. salad dressing added)
1 sliced tomato
carrot stick

Mid afternoon
1 ounce hard cheddar cheese

Supper
filet of sole (broiled) (6 oz.)
spinach
1 boiled potato
tea or coffee with milk

1000 Calories

Breakfast
1 cup apricot nectar
bran flakes (¾ cup)
1 cup whole milk
(sugar substitute may be
    added for sweetening)
coffee or tea with milk

Mid morning
small apple

Lunch
salad (lettuce, tomato,
    cucumber, celery,
    radishes with one tbsp. oil
    and vinegar dressing)
½ cup cottage cheese
coffee or tea with milk

Mid afternoon
1 cup V-8 juice

Supper
2 slices fried calves liver
boiled potato
Brussels sprouts
1 cup fresh strawberries
coffee or tea with milk

1500 Calories

Breakfast
½ cup unsweetened orange
    juice
2 scrambled eggs (cooked in
    spray-on shortening)
½ broiled tomato
1 slice whole wheat toast
    with pat of butter
coffee or tea with milk

Mid morning
1 banana

Lunch
1 cup consomme
tuna salad (3 oz. tuna, cel-
    ery, 1 tsp. salad dressing)
2 olives
tomatoes, cucumber slices
1 wedge melon

Mid afternoon
1 cup V-8 juice
1 ounce cheddar cheese

Supper
baked potato with topping
(1 tsp. sour cream, or 1
tsp. butter)
2 broccoli spears
broiled steak (3 oz.)

Late snack
½ cup of grapefruit, orange,
and apple chunks

1500 Calories

Breakfast
½ grapefruit
1 breakfast sausage link
4 cherry tomatoes
1 poached egg
coffee or tea with milk

Mid morning
bran muffin
coffee or tea with milk

Lunch
New England clam chowder
celery and carrot sticks
1 tomato sliced
1 apple

Mid afternoon
½ cup cottage cheese

Supper
V-8 juice
roast beef (3 oz.)
green peas
carrots
baked potato with pat of
butter
½ cantaloupe

Late snack
1 ounce cheddar cheese
1 glass whole milk

2000 Calories

Breakfast
½ cup orange juice (un-
   sweetened)
oatmeal with milk
2 poached eggs
1 slice rye bread with pat of
   butter
coffee or tea with milk

Mid morning
1 cup V-8 juice

Lunch
1 cup split pea soup
2 ounces cheese (mild
   Gouda)
1 slice whole wheat bread
   with pat of butter

Mid afternoon
1 banana

Supper
1 lamb chop (4.8 oz. with
   bone)
½ cup brown rice
green beans with mush-
   rooms
carrots
1 cup fresh blueberries with
   cream

Late snack
½ cup egg custard

2000 Calories

Breakfast
1 cup V-8 juice
2 strips bacon
2 egg omelet (cooked in
   spray-on shortening)
tea or coffee with milk
toast/butter

Mid morning
1 apple
coffee or tea with milk

Lunch
cream of mushroom soup
Greek salad (lettuce, to-
   matoes, feta cheese,
   black olives, oil and
   vinegar dressing)
1 orange
coffee or tea with milk

Mid afternoon
1 ounce cheddar cheese
tea or coffee with milk

Supper
pork chop (3 oz. broiled)
cabbage/carrots
baked potato with topping
    (1 tsp. sour cream or but-
    ter)
strawberries (with plain yo-
    gurt)
coffee or tea with milk

Late snack
1 glass whole milk
1 biscuit (Arrowroot)

2,500 Calories

Breakfast
½ melon
2 scrambled eggs (Cooked
    in spray-on shortening)
breakfast sausages (2)
1 slice whole wheat toast
    with butter
1 tsp. honey
coffee or tea with milk

Mid morning
5 oz. fruit yogurt

Lunch
1 cup consommé
salmon salad
tomatoes, celery, cucumber
French bread/butter

Mid afternoon
2 ounces cheddar cheese
4 cherry tomatoes

Supper
shrimp cocktail (4 oz.) with
    sauce
broiled New York sirloin
    steak
baked potato with pat of
    butter
green beans with sauteed
    mushrooms
carrots
1 cup fresh raspberries

Late snack
1 cup vanilla ice cream

2,500 Calories

Breakfast
orange juice
1 cup Special K with milk
and sugar
1 egg boiled
2 slices bacon
1 piece whole wheat toast
with butter
coffee or tea with milk

Mid morning
2 ounces cheddar cheese
1 Arrowroot biscuit
coffee or tea with milk

Lunch
1 cup V-8 juice
corned beef (4 oz.)
1 slice rye bread with pat of
butter
green salad with oil and
vinegar dressing
½ cup egg custard
½ pear

Mid afternoon
blender drink made with 2
tbsp. milk and egg protein
powder, banana, 1 tsp of
vanilla, 1 tsp honey, 1 cup
whole milk

Supper
onion soup with parmesan
cheese
broiled salmon
asparagus
carrots
boiled potato
¼ cup white sauce (thin)
fresh peaches with yogurt

Late snack
1 glass whole milk

3,000 Calories

Breakfast
1 glass grapefruit juice
oatmeal with milk and 1
    tbsp. honey
2 poached eggs
3 strips bacon
1 slice whole wheat
    bread/butter
coffee or tea with milk

Mid morning
6 oz. fruit flavored yogurt
coffee or tea with milk

Lunch
1 cup tomato juice
green salad with dressing
sirloin steak (3 oz.)
mashed potato
corn
sauteed mushrooms
1 cup fresh pineapple
    chunks

Mid afternoon
banana
1 glass whole milk with 1
    tbsp. protein added

Supper
pea soup
roll/butter
pork chop
apple sauce
broccoli
carrots
½ cup vanilla ice cream

3,000 Calories

Breakfast
½ grapefruit (sprinkle with 1 tsp. sugar)
2 eggs scrambled (cooked in spray-on shortening)
2 oz. ham
broiled tomato
2 slices whole wheat toast with butter
1 cup whole milk
coffee or tea with milk

Mid morning
1 ounce cheddar cheese
1 apple
coffee or tea with milk

Lunch
V-8 Juice
2 oz. roast beef sandwich
small green salad with oil and vinegar dressing
1 tangerine

Mid afternoon
protein drink (milk, protein, orange juice)

Supper
3 oz. filet of sole
green beans
2 boiled potatoes with butter
egg custard with peach half

Late snack
6 oz. fruit yogurt

VITAMINS AND FOOD SUPPLEMENTS

Experts cannot say exactly what constitutes *the* perfectly balanced diet for you as an individual. Supplementing your diet with vitamins, minerals, and food supplements can be viewed as an insurance policy. If you're involved in regular exercise, you might want to take a multi-vitamin/mineral pill (the one-a-day variety). Some people supplement the pill with individual vitamins. For example, extra vitamins B, C, and E.

It's possible to overdo your intake of vitamins, minerals and other supplements. The body will simply not assimilate more than it needs and you could suffer

nausea from the toxicity caused by overdosing yourself with vitamins A or D.

**Do not take any of the items discussed in this section
without first checking with your doctor.**

Vitamin B is good for your nervous system. Vitamin
C keeps the arteries and capillaries supple, and *may*
help ward off colds. Vitamin E, *may* be partly respon-
sible for maintaining proper hormone levels.

People frequently insist that added supplements are
unnecessary. However many people, including trained
athletes, are often found to be deficient in vitamins and
minerals when tested. Many women are deficient in
iron. If you suspect this applies to you because you are
constantly tired, see your doctor. He may advise you
to take extra iron.

Some people believe in taking a protein powder as
an additive in addition to vitamins. There are many
brands to be found at health food stores. Most are
made from soya beans, milk or milk and egg. The percentage of protein usually varies from 40% to 90%.

Protein powders are often taken by athletes who
need added strength, muscle size, or who need to gain
weight. They can be mixed with milk, fruit or yogurt.
Ironically, protein powders can also be used to aid in
weight *loss*. Instead of adding them to a three or four
meal regime (as you would if you wanted to gain
weight), you should mix the protein supplement with
juice instead of milk, and take it as a meal *substitute*.
In other words, you would drop one meal and take a
protein mix instead.

X

POWERLIFTING

Women who want to take up the sport of *powerlifting* should remember that it is a competitive sport. The objective is to lift the most weight in any of the following categories: *squat lift,* the *bench press* and the *dead lift.* Most women currently competing (and there are hundreds in the States alone) do so because they have a husband, brother, or boyfriend who are *into* powerlifting. The ladies are usually cajoled into it at first, and once hooked—that's it! They love it. There are a few powerlift meets specifically for women, but mostly, as in marathon running, the ladies compete alongside the men. In some cases the women are coming out on top. I believe that women will dominate powerlifting in all but the bench press, in the near future. The "weaker" sex have *very* strong backs, hips and legs and both the squat and the dead lift require real strength in these areas. I base my prediction on this anatomical fact.

If you want to become a powerlifter, you must have

a basic foundation of overall strength and conditioning. If you follow the training schedules mentioned you will be properly prepared.

No one, male or female, should start training for powerlifting contests without at least six months of general all-around weight workouts.

When you decide you have gained sufficient strength and power to train for competition, the wisest thing to do is join a "heavy duty" gym. This is a gym with apparatus like Olympic bars, squat racks, power stands and extra heavy benches.

Pick a gym whose members are dedicated weight lifters, who are interested in improving their abilities. The friendly rivalry and infectious atmosphere of enthusiastic lifters will motivate you and your strength will increase more rapidly than if you were training at home.

Here are the official rules of The International Federation of Body Builders for the three basic lifts:

Squat Lift

1. Lifter shall stand upright with bar in horizontal position across shoulders.
2. Toes shall be placed touching actual or imaginary straight line.
3. Feet spacing shall be optional.
4. Heel wedges, if used, shall not exceed 2 inches in height.
5. All forms of wrapping, cushioning, taping or bandaging of any part of the legs shall be disallowed.
6. Padding may be applied only to the bar and shall not exceed 12 inches in width or two inches at its thickest point.

7. The bar shall be held in place with the hands and shall not be lower than one inch below the highest part of the deltoid.

8. Method of bringing the bar to the shoulders in preparation for the lift shall be optional.

9. The lifter shall await the referee's signal in a controlled and steady position, facing front.

10. At the signal, the lifter shall lower the body, bending the knees, bringing the center of the thighs below, parallel with the floor.

11. Lifter shall then regain the upright position without bouncing or undue hesitation until his knees are fully locked back and still. Lifter must remain in this position until the referee signals his approval.

12. All apparatus used shall meet American standards.

13. Judges and referees shall have an unobscured view of the lift at all times.

Rules for disqualification

1. Failure to obey referee's signals.

2. Raising of heels or toes, change of position of hands or feet during lift.

3. Bouncing of either weight or knees.

4. More than one attempt at recovery to the upright position.

5. Failure to make the upright "lock back" knee position or hold same at the start or completion of lift.

6. Any movement of the bar during lift.

7. Any touching or interference with the bar by the spotters before the referee's approval.

Bench Press

1. The "bench" shall not be less than 10 inches nor more than 23 inches in width; and not less than 14 inches nor more than 18 inches in height.
2. Either of the two following positions may be adopted by the lifter, but once adopted, maintained throughout the lift:

    a) Entire body extended in a flat "knees locked" supine position on the bench.

    b) Head, body (including buttocks) resting on supine bench with feet resting flat on the floor (should lifter's feet not reach comfortably to the floor, resting, blocks shall be allowed).
3. The distance between the lifter's hands shall not exceed 32 inches between index fingers.
4. Lifter's apparel shall contrast enough in color and/or tone with the bench top, so as to make any possible raising or movement of the buttocks apparent to the judges.
5. The lifter shall await referee's signal to commence lift with the bar resting motionless on the chest.
6. Method of bringing bar to the starting position (5) shall be at the discretion of the lifter.
7. At the referee's signal the lifter shall raise the bar vertically to the straight arm position where it must remain in a controlled steady position until the referee signals the lift is completed.
8. Judges and referees shall have an unobscured view of the lift at all times.
9. A minimum of two safety spotters shall be in attendance.

Rules for disqualification

1. Failure to obey referee's signals.
2. Bracing feet or shoulders against bench or bench uprights.
3. Contacting uprights during the lift.
4. All forms of wrapping, cushioning, taping or bandaging any part of the body shall be disallowed.
5. Change or interchange of lifting position.
6. Lifting or raising of legs, shoulders, buttocks, hips, head or feet during the lift.
7. Any movement of the above.
8. Bridging of the body.
9. Bouncing the bar from or on the chest.
10. Resting bar on the chest.
11. Allowing the bar to sink unduly into the chest or stomach.
12. Stopping or jerking the bar's progress during the lift.
13. Unlevel extension of the arms.
14. Any touching or interference with the bar by the spotters before the referee's approval.

Deadlift

1. The lifter shall position himself ready to attempt the lift and await the referee's signal.
2. Lifter shall have optional grip with both hands and leg spacing.
3. Bar shall be placed horizontal in front of lifter's feet.
4. From the bent position the lifter must stand upright lifting the weight in one continuous movement until standing in an erect knees lock position with shoulders thrust back.

5. Judges and referees shall have an unobscured view of the lift at all times.
6. The upright position must be held in a controlled and steady fashion until the referee signals his approval.

Rules for disqualification
1. Failure to obey referee's signals.
2. Stopping or hesitation of the bar during the lift.
3. Failure to regain the upright position with knees locked.
4. Resting the bar on the thighs.
5. More than one attempt.
6. Movement of feet during the lift.
7. Raising of the heels or toes.

Training for competition can take many forms. Generally the best results come from a schedule in which each lift is practiced twice a week.

When training to improve your strength in power lifts obviously you must actually practice those lifts. However, after a few months of training exclusively on each movement, it's a good idea to add supplementary exercises to strengthen any weak links.

Your squat schedule may look like this:

Squat (warm-up)	1 × 12
Squat (adding weight each set)	1 × 5
	2 × 4
	2 × 3
	2 × 2

A supplementary exercise

¼ squat (much heavier weight)	1 × 6
Add weight each set	4 × 2

Your bench press schedule
Bench Press (forearms vertical)
(warm up)   1 × 12
Bench press (adding weight each set)   2 × 6
                                             2 × 4
                                             4 × 2

A supplementary exercise
Dumbell bench press (add weight each set)   1 × 6
                                             4 × 2

Dead lift schedule
Dead lift (warm up)   1 × 12
Dead lift (adding weight each set)   1 × 6
                                             2 × 4
                                             2 × 3
                                             1 × 2

Supplementary exercise
Partial deadlifts from low supports (or
boxes)   1 × 6
Add weight each set   3 × 3
                                             1 × 2

It is a good idea to find a coach if you are serious about powerlifting. Many gyms have accomplished instructors who are only too willing to help out with training advice. Once you have decided to put your trust in a coach, then follow his or her instructions to the letter. Nothing is more annoying to a dedicated coach than to give his time to help an athlete reach her peak, only to find that she's not following his advice. Listen only to your coach. By all means talk things over with him (or her) but do not listen to the hundred and one know-it-alls who will proffer "advice" left, right and center. Usually they will not know as much as your coach, and their advice is seldom backed by scientific knowledge.

As a powerlifter you should read the two main weight training magazines that deal with powerlifting techniques.

Muscular Development
P.O. Box 1707
York, Pa. 17405

Iron Man Magazine
Box 10
Alliance, Nebraska 69301

As you advance you will find that your schedule will alter slightly from workout to workout. Sometimes your strength is "up." Sometimes it's "down." This is natural. The body has its good days and its bad days. Sometimes your normal exercise poundage feels pretty good, almost light. On other days, and for no obvious reason, your weights feel like a ton. What should you do? Just do your best. If you can't "lift" your regular weights, be satisfied with less weight. However, on the days when your weights feel light, take advantage of the moment. Pile on a little more and you'll probably be stronger for future workouts.

Entering your first powerlift contest can be a memorable occasion. Unless you have super strength, I suggest you enter a local meet rather than one of state or national status. Then you won't feel too nervous about the competition. You will find contests advertised in *Muscular Development* magazine, on Y.M.C.A. bulletin boards, and on the notice boards of some "heavy duty" gyms. The notices always give an address to write to for "entry" forms. The usual forms ask your name, address, sex, and number of years in training— little more. Nothing personal. You will be notified when to arrive. You will find that weights are supplied backstage where you and the other contestants can warm-up. Take care not to warm-up too soon before "lifting." As the time approaches, listen carefully for your name to be called out for your first lift. Needless to say you should know your lifting capacity and strength and be able to judge the correct poundage for each lift. You get three attempts at each. You can increase the weight whenever you try a lift, but you are not permitted to call for *less* weight than you attempted on your prior effort.

All time best lifts for women (as of Jan. 1979)

114 lbs. Class	Squat	Bench Press	Dead Lift	Total
Terry Dillard	255 lbs.	110 lbs.	315 lbs.	680 lbs.
Sheila Hopkins	215	120	300	635
Sue Elwyn	195	145	245	585
Linda Madzey	205	120	260	585
Terry Poston	210	125	240	575
Pam Meister	205	95	275	575
Cheryl Daniels	205	115	225	545
Charlene Fanny	190	110	245	545
Shirley Patterson	185	120	225	530
Stella Martinez	185	110	230	525
Cheryl Jackson	180	85	210	475
Kathy Parsons	140	95	210	445
Jodi Seigel	155	90	175	420
Mary Tanner	145	75	200	420
Darlene Veinot	140	65	205	410
Becky Chapman	100	55	225	380
Cheryl Adams	125	75	175	375
Gail Goldstein	85	65	175	325
Sandy Fautersack	170	85	255	510
123 lb. Class				
Sheila Hopkins	215	125	305	645
Karen Hofmeyer	225	105	290	620

Susan Johnson	190	125	270	585
Carol Stuhlatz	205	95	270	570
Natalie Kahn	170	105	250	525
Darlene Linhart	155	90	225	470
Naomi Handa	150	95	225	470
Dee Ann Peters	150	90	215	455
Judy Waterman	150	90	210	450
Cathy Nelson	140	85	220	445
Kathy Melcher	140	90	210	440
Kathy Kestel	155	75	170	400
Valerie Rafuse	105	75	190	370
Shelley Farber	105	95	165	365
Carolyn Reid	115	90	135	340
Pam Jacobson	180	115	255	550

132 lb. Class

Becky Joubert	260	155	340	755
Jeanna French	230	120	300	650
Beverly Cook	195	125	270	590
Jan Irwin	210	110	260	580
Mary Nelson	205	115	260	580
Dorie McArthur	185	105	250	540
Sue Hommertzheim	200	105	220	525
Natalie Kahn	165	105	210	480
Doreen Tracey	155	85	210	450
Marilyn Skerback	145	100	200	445
Darlene Wamback	160	80	205	445
Tammy Harmon	155	85	195	435
Ann Eagles	155	80	160	395
Marge Aseltyne	135	75	175	385
Toni D'Errico	135	75	175	385
Sue Gaye	95	80	200	375

148 lb. Class

Becky Joubert	270	165	355	790
Kathy Copp	275	180	295	750
Julie McEwen	210	145	325	680
Cindy Groffman	275	105	270	650
Dena Lowe	145	85	225	455

148 lb. Class

Carla Jo Kuhnen	155	85	205	445
Debbie Langevain	250	135	335	720
Karin Smith	220	145	335	700
Jeanne St. Pierre	250	135.	335	720
Susan Jones	260	120	290	670
Angela Lassa	240	100	265	605

165 lb. Class

Beverley Francis	319	225	363	907
Ann Turbyne	345	210	400	955
Cindy Reinhoudt	355	215	380	980
Ann Turbyne	320	180	410	910
Stephanie Moody	335	180	385	900
Cheryl Waltz	250	170	300	720
Julie McEwen	185	135	320	640
Linda Clark	165	115	275	555
Rosa Quintero	175	125	200	500
Donna Carter	170	90	240	500

181 lb. Class

Jan Todd	375	175	451	1001
Cindy Reinhoudt	370	210	385	965
Barbara Burns	205	80	240	525
Loraine Rothman	145	100	220	465

Unlimited Class

Jan Todd	424	176	441	1041
Jennifer Burgess	135	80	230	445
Debra Blomley	125	80	230	435

Only experience will teach you what poundage to select. If for example your best bench press is 110 lbs, call for 100 lbs in your first attempt, 110 pounds for your second, and if successful, a third record attempt of 120 lbs. Who knows one day you may become a winner!

XI

QUESTIONS AND ANSWERS

Q   I know this may sound like a silly question but I am concerned and would like to know the truth. Does weight training (a) Damage the heart? (b) Cause one to become musclebound? (c) Shorten one's lifespan?

A *(a)* If your heart is normal, then progressive resistance exercise will do nothing but good. Your heart is a very powerful muscle and as such, like your other muscles, requires stimulation to keep it strong and healthy.

    (b) Perhaps the greatest single misconception about weight training is that it will cause one to become "musclebound." Actually there are few things quite as pliable, supple or elastic as muscle. Consequently people who exercise cor-

rectly with weights enjoy better coordination, flexibility and agility than the average non-athletic person. In weight training you should always completely contract and extend your muscles during each exercise. This will not give you normal flexibility. It will give you *superior* flexibility. To put that another way, instead of becoming "musclebound," you will become just the opposite.

(c) Your lifespan is governed initially by your genes. If you come from a family which tends to live to a "ripe old age" then you have a head start. The other aids to living a long healthy life are principally up to you. Proper nutrition is important. Uncontrolled eating, drinking, smoking, and pill taking may reduce your lifespan. Vigorous exercise such as weight training is a *plus* because exercise is necessary to help maintain heart, lung and muscular efficiency, all of which contributes to good health and longevity.

Q I once lifted my boyfriend's barbells for just a couple of minutes. The next day I could hardly move. I had aching, sore muscles for a week. I can't bear the thought of this happening again.

A Anytime one subjects one's body to a new form of exercise there will be *some* soreness. If you want to avoid this, do not use weights that put a severe demand on your unexercised muscles. Start with just the bar. Gradually, as you get used to the exertion, you will be able to add weights to the bar. Start weight training *slowly* and you will avoid excessive soreness.

Q I get the occasional urge to diet and exercise but I always give up within a couple of days. Any suggestions?

A I suppose it's a matter of motivation. Talk yourself into staying with your workouts. *You* know you want to improve your body. You know that doing *nothing* will only make you more discontent as each day passes and you become less energetic and less shapely. Ask yourself this: "Is it too much to give a couple of hours a week to molding yourself into a million dollar package of femininity?" To be successful at anything set your mind to it! That's the only way to accomplish even a modicum of success. If your mind is lazy, then your body will respond accordingly. If your mind is active, energetic and lively your body will reflect it. Success or failure can be attributed to mental attitude. With practice and determination you can increase your drive. Working out regularly will in itself cement and increase your self discipline and will power. Program your mind for success today!

Q Will I develop callouses if I exercise with weights?

A Yes, long workouts with barbells may form callouses at the base of the fingers on the underside of the hands, as may rowing, canoeing, biking and numerous other sports. You can avoid this by wearing thin gloves whenever you train.

Q I am pregnant and everybody is trying to make me take it easy. I feel like being active. Is there any reason not to exercise vigorously during pregnancy?

A Generally speaking, there is no reason to reduce your activity during the first months of pregnancy. Obviously, really heavy sports or contact games are out, but many women are finding that moderately strenuous exercise right up until the last month of pregnancy can be very beneficial. The key here of course, is to consult your doctor, because he may possibly be aware of some underlying reason why you personally should not indulge in vigorous exercise.

Q I weigh 105 pounds at 5′9″ height, and my doctor has recommended that I take up weight lifting to gain weight. But I have a further problem: I have large veins running up and down my legs and arms. They are not varicose veins, but I don't want to make them worse and I am afraid weights will bring them out even more.

A Veins are inherited and only show on the surface when there is virtually no fat covering the outer layer of the body. Your present weight is far too low for your height. Your doctor is right. As a further aid, I suggest you increase your calorie intake significantly. In this way you will gradually hide your protruding veins with a slight covering of adipose tissue.

Q I have always enjoyed long distance running. My husband and I run about 50 miles a week. Is there any reason why I should not do weight training in addition to my running?

A Weight training will strengthen and shape muscles that running does not. It may be wise to introduce your weight training very slowly and perhaps reduce your weekly running distance, at least until your body has gotten used to the increased energy and recuperative demands. If you feel drained and washed out the day after, then it is likely that you will have to reduce your overall exercise program. Be guided by moderation in all things rather than allow your enthusiasm to draw you into overtiring yourself, and possibly losing interest altogether.

Q   If I take up regular weight training to shape up my body, what happens when I stop? Will I become flabby? Are there any dangers in suddenly stopping a vigorous exercise program?

A   No, no, no. After the Olympic games literally tens of thousands of athletes stop training. Most get back to it because they have learned to love strenuous activity, but there are no automatic ill-effects to curtailing heavy exercise. What you will notice after stopping is that you have an abundance of energy, especially when your normal workout time comes around. Neither will you automatically get fat. What usually happens when all exercise is stopped, is that the body tends to *slowly* revert to its original state. In other words, if you were fat *before* starting an exercise program then you will slowly become fat again. If you were thin, then you will become thin again, all things being equal. Bear in mind that your food intake is always of prime importance where weight is concerned. A good example would be a boxer who must train heavily for a match, and eat heftily to fill his energy requirements. After the match, when he is no longer running, skipping, and sparring, if he

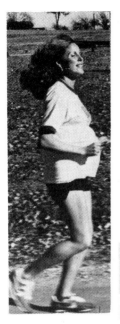

Mary Jones, of Dallas, Texas, like many other physical fitness buffs, jogs about 40 miles a week. She ran through her last two pregnancies and quit three weeks before the baby was born. She resumed three weeks after the birth.

Jacqueline Robichaud, of Mississauga, Ontario, has placed high in the Annual Miss Canada contest. Here she demonstrates an exercise for the entire tummy area.

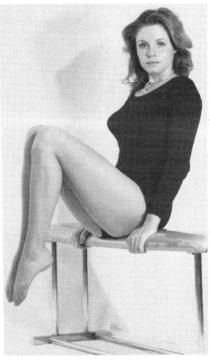

continues to eat as he did during training, rather than burning up those calories with vigorous exercise, he will store them as—fat! If you drastically alter or limit *your* physical activities, then also reduce the amount you eat. In this way you will be able to control your weight to the pound.

Q   The lower part of my stomach sticks out. I have tried situps for the last three months but just cannot lose this ugly lower pot belly. What do you suggest?

A   Situps do not work the lower part of the stomach. In fact, they exercise the muscles of the upper tummy area near the chest. Try hanging knee raises instead. Hang on a horizontal bar (a doorway gym bar is ideal) and raise both knees up as near to the chin as you can get them. Try "sets" of ten to fifteen repetitions every day. This will firm up the sagging muscles. If you are also overweight, exercise alone is not the answer. You will have to combine this exercise with fewer calories.

Q   Are there any vitamins or special foods I can take to lose fat and firm up?

A   Although grapefruit is a favorite with dieters, it probably has no special fat destroying properties. However, many beauty contestants take a variety of supplements which they claim helps to maintain a lean, fat-free appearance. Some are listed below but check first with your doctor.

1. *Choline and Inositol* (Available from your

drug store, non-prescription) This is a concentrated fat emulsifier.

2. *Kelp tablets* (health food store) The iodine content is supposed to speed up metabolism.
3. *Thyroxine* (A prescription drug) Available only from your doctor if your metabolism is too slow.
4. *Vitamin C* (health food store) Firms loose skin and rebuilds cells.
5. *Protein powder* (health food store) Substitutes for a meal. The protein is there with a minimum of fat and other ingredients. (Protein uses *more* energy than other foods when being digested.)

Q I am 5′6″ in height, weigh 146 but I am *not* fat. Every part of my body is firm muscle. I can understand that exercise and diet can reduce superfluous flab, but how on earth am I going to reduce all this muscle? I am definitely too heavy and big.

A I suspect that you probably have a large bone structure and that nature blessed (?) you with long, full muscles to go with the bones.

Please bear in mind that different Western societies and cultures have varied ideas of what constitutes a perfect female physique.

In the high fashion world of London and Paris the extremely thin, hollow chested, flat breasted, poorly postured body is considered tops.

In modern beauty contests, the firm, strong bodied woman with moderately slim legs and fuller bustline is preferred.

In the athletic arenas, heavier, more muscular women have set a new standard of near Amazonian perfection.

The point is, of course, nature does not always accommodate your preferences. If you don't fit the category that appeals to you most, it is because you had no choice. You were born with your type of body.

However, a woman with a large skeletal structure *can* reduce her muscle size, through a daily exercise regimen which should probably include up to ten minutes of skipping (or half an hour of jogging) *plus* a strict diet. Just as a fat body deprived of food will "eat" its own fat reserve, so will a heavily muscled body "starved" of calories also *reduce* in size. Energy requirements have to be filled first and your body will rob both fat and muscle reserves to meet these fundamental demands.

Q   What is meant by the term "empty" calories?

A   "Empty" calories are energy (calories) that one ingests from food which is otherwise nutritionally useless. Common examples include chocolate bars, sugar, candies, synthetic cookies, colas and cakes. You could form a diet around these items and still keep within your daily calorie plan, but your health would suffer since you would not be getting the correct vitamins, minerals, proteins etc.

Q   How do I firm up the outside of my thighs?

A   This is a problem with many women. The upper outer areas of their thighs have a pad of fatty flesh that shows not only in a swimsuit but also in jeans and even in a dress. There are exercises that put stress on this particular area exclusively, such as the side leg raise: Lie on the floor (on your side) and raise your uppermost leg towards the ceiling. Work up to twenty repetitions. Exercise both legs equally by turning over and raising the other leg. However, the problem requires not only exercise, but also a change of diet. It is probably best to follow an overall body conditioning program which includes leg exercises, and to follow a controlled diet.

Q I am on the thin side, and to make matters worse I have small breasts. To be frank my chest is pretty flat. Please help.

A Exercises such as the bench press will work the pectoralis muscles of the upper chest. This in turn will tend to raise and firm the area. But the breasts themselves are not influenced by exercises. They do not grow bigger since they are glandular rather than muscular in nature. Of course, there is a tendency for the overall bustline measurement to increase as one gains weight. Also, both pregnancy and the pill tend to increase bustline size. This may not make one iota of difference to your anxiety, but most men (*men,* not boys) do not require that women have large breasts. They are more turned on by fat free, trim bodies than large mammary glands. Also, there's a growing army of men who actually prefer women with small shapely breasts.

Q My problem is losing weight. I diet very strictly and exercise regularly but in spite of greatly limiting my carbohydrate intake, I just cannot lose weight. Is my problem glandular?

A   Don't count carbohydrates, calories are what you should be counting. Overweight due to glandular irregularities is relatively rare, but if there is any doubt, see your doctor. Unfortunately, people who have been overweight for a long time, or since childhood, may find it impossible to lose *all* their superfluous fat. And some people have a *slight* metabolic defect—a low rate of burning energy while the body is at rest. Again your doctor is the one to consult. If he suspects your metabolism is out of kilter he may recommend a nutritional expert, or treat you himself. Exercise on a regular basis can stimulate one's metabolic rate.

Q   I have read about the by-pass operation for losing weight. Please tell me what it is exactly.

A   The by-pass procedure is a full-fledged operation whereby a surgeon removes a length of your intestines. Because some people pass food through this area slowly the body has more time to extract calories from the food and consequently these people tend to be heavier than others whose systems are speedier. Exercise is often recommended for this state of near constipation. The by-pass operation is the most extreme treatment for chronically overweight people, and is not recommended at all for the average overweight person.

Q   In addition to situps and leg raises, could you please indicate a further exercise that will work the front part of my waistline. I have a flabby tummy and just about no underlying firmness to my lower abdominal area.

A Try bench leg raises: Sit on bench, hands holding the sides. Lean back and raise your legs as shown in the photograph. While keeping knees bent, lower and raise the legs, endeavoring to touch the knees to the chest. Try 2 sets of 15 after your regular workout.

FURTHER READING

Barrilleaux, Doris, and Murray, Jim. *Inside Weight Training for Women*. Chicago: Contemporary Books Inc., 1978.

Carnes, Valerie and Ralph. *Body Sculpture: Weight Training for Women*. New York: Simon and Schuster, 1978.

Columbu, Drs. Anita and Franco. *Star Bodies*. New York: E. P. Dutton, 1979.

Davis, Ellen. *Bodybuilding for Women*. Self-published, 1978.

Heidenstam, Oscar. *Modern Bodybuilding*. Buchanan, N.Y.: Emerson Books, Inc., 1970.

Modern Health and Figure Culture. London: Faber and Faber, 1960.

Kennedy, Robert. *Shape-Up*. New York: Frederick Fell, 1978.

Lance, Kathryn. *Getting Strong*. Indianapolis: The Bobbs-Merrill Company, Inc., 1978.

Randall, Bruce. *The Barbell Way to Physical Fitness*. New York: Doubleday, 1970.

Ravelle, Lou. *Bodybuilding for Everyone*. Buchanan, N.Y.: Emerson Books, Inc., 1965.

Reynolds, Bill. *Complete Weight Training*. Mountainview, Ca.: World Publications, 1976.

Schwarzenegger, Arnold. *Arnold: The Education of a Bodybuilder*. New York: Simon and Schuster, 1977.

Sing, Vanessa. *Lift for Life*. New York: Bolder Books, 1976.

Sprague, Ken. *Gold's Gym Weight Training Book for a Beautiful, Strong, Healthy Body*. New York: St. Martin's Press, 1978.

Zane, Christine. *The Feminine Physique: Bodybuilding for the Woman*. Self published, 1978.

Zane, Christine and Frank. *The Zane Way to a Beautiful Body*. New York: Simon and Schuster, 1979.

Magazines

Feminine Muscularity, "Specializing in Well-Formed Training for Women", T.R. Puryear, Box 16, Station B, Long Branch, N.J. 07740.

Iron Man, 512 Blackhills Ave., Alliance, Ne 69301.

Muscle Builder/Power, "Covering the Bodybuilding Field", 21100 Erwin St., Woodland Hills, CA 91364.

Muscle Mag International, "Dedicated to the Survival of the Fittest", P.O. Box 2009, Bramalea, Ontario, Canada L6T 3S3.

Vital, "The Magazine for Healthy Living", 1201 Kirk St., Elk Grove Village, IL 60007

CONTESTS

Not everyone reading this book will want to enter a physical excellence (or beauty) contest, but it is a way of gauging your progress. Besides, it can be fun. Win or lose you will probably enjoy the experience. And besides, when you enter a few of these contests, you will find a whole new world of friends and acquaintances. There are literally thousands of different beauty contests held throughout the North American and European contest circuit.

Because of the prestige of some contests and the financial rewards as well, many women travel throughout North America and even to Europe. You will find many of these women's bodybuilding contests advertised under *coming events* in *Muscular Development* magazine (Box 1707, York, Pa. 17405) and Joe Weider's *Muscle Builder/Power* magazine (21100 Erwin St., Woodland Hills, CA., 91364).

In addition the annual *Miss Bikini* contest in London, England, is run every September by publisher and physical culture expert Oscar Heidenstam. Entry forms can be obtained by writing Oscar at: 30 Craven St., Strand, London, WC2N 5NT, England. Send $1 to cover mailing costs.

Show organizer George Snyder of the Olympus Gym Spa, Warrington, Pa., has formed the Women's Bodybuilding Association (WBA) and he runs numerous physical excellence contests for female bodybuilders. Further information on this association and any women's contests run by the Olympus Health Spa can be had by writing to George Snyder, Rt. 611, Warrington, Pa. 18976.

In New York every fall impressario Dan Lurie runs the *Miss Body Beautiful* contest in conjunction with his annual *Mr. Olympus* contest. Entry forms can be obtained by applying to Dan Lurie Barbell Co., 1665 Utica Ave., Brooklyn, N.Y., 11234.

When entering a women's contest there are a few things to note in preparation:

1. Turn up on time for the pre-judging. Most contests are actually judged in the morning; the evening show is the performance that the public pays to see.
2. Make sure you have an even tan. If you have not been able to get this naturally from the sun, then apply it the night before with several layers of instant tanning lotion.
3. Practice your posing. Each woman is expected to walk to center stage, step up onto a simple podium and run through a brief routine of poses to show off her figure.
4. Contest preparation cannot be done at the last minute. Prepare your body as completely as you

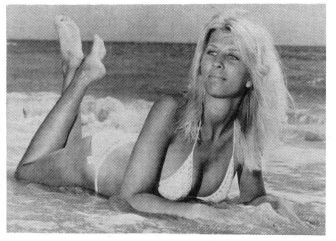

Pat Young, of Miami Beach, was voted Florida's most photo-graphic girl by Florida's pressmen.

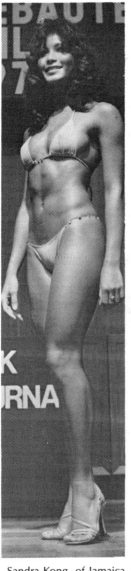
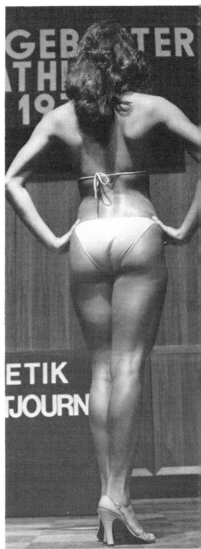

Sandra Kong, of Jamaica, shows what intelligent progressive resistance training can accomplish.

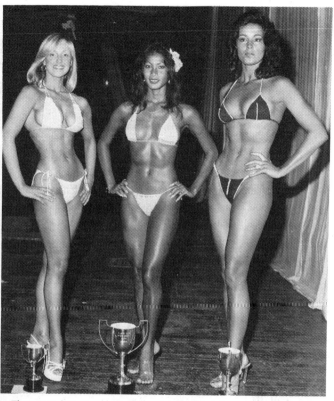

Three top beauty contestants who took top honors in the prestigious NABBA Miss Bikini Contest. (Left to Right: Bridget Gibbons,
3rd, Sandra Kong, 1st, and Linda Cheeseman, 2nd.) All are into
vigorous weight training.

can prior to the day of competition. If you are carrying a small amount of superfluous weight then go on a diet three weeks before the event. Some women who want to be excessively lean for contests eat only fish, grapefruit juice and water during the last three days before the contest. Limit your liquids as the day of the contest approaches.

5. Select a costume that is suited to your particular figure. Some big pageants, especially those televised, insist on all the women wearing identically-styled swim costumes. However, for the most part the swim garment you wear on the big night is *your* choice. Costumes with high cut sides make the thighs look longer. Whether or not you wear a two-piece or a one-piece is up to your judgment of your figure. Again, a few contests stipulate which are to be born. For example, all women who enter the *Nabba Miss Bikini* in England are required to wear bikinis.

6. Select shoes that complement your legs. High heels are desirable, but do not select heels so high or precarious that you appear awkward when walking, or are in danger of tottering over.

7. Make sure your posture is as perfect as possible. Smile and practice looking as confident as you are able so that you will not look nervous (even if you are).

8. Finally, win or lose, show that you are big hearted on the night. Accept your trophy graciously if you are lucky enough to win and bear with the fans and legions of photographers. Should you not take the top award, offer the winner your congratulations and above all keep smiling.

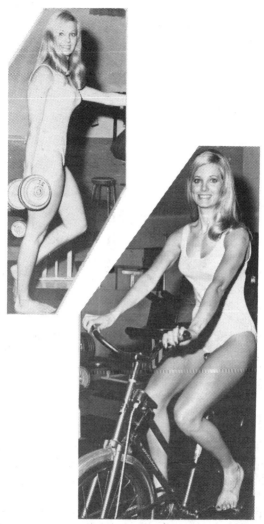

Toni Chellew, of South Africa, is every inch a bodybuilder. She trains with weights three times a week and is now winning physical excellence contests. (Photo: Kallos)

FINALE
The end of this book;
the beginning of you

Remember, you only get out of this program what you are prepared to put into it. We all want something for nothing, or for less effort than it takes. But if it were that easy, we would all have perfect bodies. And one only has to look around to see that very few people indeed have perfect bodies.

But if you stay with it, if you rearrange your eating habits in accordance with our suggestions, work out every other day, and keep at it—results will materialize before your very eyes!

If you want that body badly enough, nothing can stop you. Your enthusiasm will carry you through your workouts, and with that miraculous "high" only the truly eager aspirant knows, you will reach out for your goal and . . . you *will* succeed. My best wishes are with you in your efforts. Success is ahead.